# Technopharmacology

# IN SEARCH OF MEDIA

Timon Beyes, Mercedes Bunz, and Wendy Hui Kyong Chun,
Series Editors

# Technopharmacology

Joshua Neves, Aleena Chia,
Susanna Paasonen, and Ravi Sundaram

**IN SEARCH OF MEDIA**

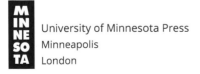
University of Minnesota Press
Minneapolis
London

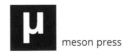
meson press

In Search of Media is a collaboration between the University
of Minnesota Press and meson press, an open access
publisher, https://meson.press.

Published by the University of Minnesota Press, 2022
111 Third Avenue South, Suite 290
Minneapolis, MN 55401-2520
https://www.upress.umn.edu

in collaboration with
meson press
Salzstrasse 1
21335 Lüneburg, Germany
https://meson.press

ISBN 978-1-5179-1415-8 (pb)
Library of Congress record available at
https://lccn.loc.gov/2021062873.

# Contents

# Series Foreword

"Media determine our situation," Friedrich Kittler infamously wrote in his Introduction to *Gramophone, Film, Typewriter*. Although this dictum is certainly extreme—and media archaeology has been critiqued for being overly dramatic and focused on technological developments—it propels us to keep thinking about media as setting the terms for which we live, socialize, communicate, organize, do scholarship, et cetera. After all, as Kittler continued in his opening statement almost thirty years ago, our situation, "in spite or because" of media, "deserves a description." What, then, are the terms—the limits, the conditions, the periods, the relations, the phrases—of media? And, what is the relationship between these terms and determination? This book series, *In Search of Media,* answers these questions by investigating the often elliptical "terms of media" under which users operate. That is, rather than produce a series of explanatory keyword-based texts to describe media practices, the goal is to understand the conditions (the "terms") under which media is produced, as well as the ways in which media impacts and changes these terms.

Clearly, the rise of search engines has fostered the proliferation and predominance of keywords and terms. At the same time, it has changed the very nature of keywords, since now any word and pattern can become "key." Even further, it has transformed the very process of learning, since search presumes that, (a) with the right phrase, any question can be answered and (b) that the answers lie within the database. The truth, in other words, is "in there." The impact of search/media on knowledge, however, goes beyond search engines. Increasingly, disciplines—from sociology to economics, from the arts to literature—are in search of media as a way to revitalize their methods and objects of study. Our current media situation therefore seems to imply a new term, understood as temporal shifts of mediatic conditioning. Most broadly, then, this series asks: What are the terms or conditions of knowledge itself?

To answer this question, each book features interventions by two (or more) authors, whose approach to a term—to begin with: *communication, pattern discrimination, markets, remain, machine, archives, organize, action at a distance, undoing networks*—diverge and converge in surprising ways. By pairing up scholars from North America and Europe, this series also advances media theory by obviating the proverbial "ten year gap" that exists across language barriers due to the vagaries of translation and local academic customs and in order to provoke new descriptions, prescriptions, and hypotheses—to rethink and reimagine what media can and must do.

# Technology + Pharmacology

**Joshua Neves, Aleena Chia,
Susanna Paasonen, and Ravi Sundaram**

The experience of the Covid-19 pandemic has significantly
accelerated ongoing transactions between twenty-first-century
biomedical and informational technologies. The sight of hundreds
of millions worldwide submitting their bodies to experimental
vaccines suggests that the modes of human security laid out by
Michel Foucault in his Collège de France lectures may in fact have
moved into a new time-space. In his 1975–1976 lectures, titled appropriately "Society Must Be Defended," Foucault spoke about how
a set of political technologies called "biopower" initiated seamless
medical and social projects to optimize life and secure it (2004).
Biopower legitimizes periodic interventions within populations in
order to preserve the larger social body. In the early months of
the pandemic Giorgio Agamben argued that the restrictions in the
name of health security suggested a "new techno-medical despo-
tism" (2020). While Agamben's statement was widely debated at
the time, what is clear is that bodily, technological, and pharmacological rearrangements have emerged worldwide. Bifo Berardi has
similarly drawn attention to new sets of "automatisms" triggered
by the pandemic: "health automatisms, techno-mediated distancing, and psychological obsessions" (2021). More broadly, this
suggests a significant modulation of "experience": now animated by

biomedical trackers, voluntary injectables, life extension therapies, and data visualizations. At the same time, vast populations have shown themselves eager to try experimental therapies for the pandemic, while others have refused or been denied them altogether. In many ways the Covid-19 experience helps frame the title of this volume: *Technopharmacology*.

This collaborative book centers on emergent affinities between big data and big pharma, broadly conceived. It brings together two significant areas of research that, at present, do not adequately speak to one another: engagements with networked technologies, digital cultures, logistical media, and a wide range of approaches to technologized life; *and* examinations of bio-economy and biotechnologies, drugs and pharmaceuticals, and a spectrum of issues tied to the economization, reproduction, and transformation of life itself. Bridging these dynamic fields, *Technopharmacology* asks what is gained by examining media technologies in relation to pharmaceuticals and pharmacology, including embodied practices like swallowing a pill or being on social media, diagnoses of pornography or internet addiction, consciousness hacking and mundane smartness initiatives. Starting out from a critical media studies perspective, our book is a modest call to expand media theoretical inquiry by attending to the biological, neurological, and pharmacological dimensions of media. Such imbrications are found in concerns that our media technologies are drug-like, push harmful habits, and undo intimacies; the cohabitation of digital devices and drugs in practices of self-optimization, work, sex, and everyday life; the kinetic performativities shored up by platformed sociality or the mobilization of public affect; as well as critical engagements with neoliberal management, biocapital, and global "life support" systems (Vora 2015). Our interests lie in how media and drugs, both separately and together, impact and transform the affective, cognitive, and somatic capacities of bodies in ways that are completely mundane and potentially extraordinary, and that both expand and truncate capacities to thrive. Such questions are central to Susanna Paasonen's analysis of addiction and excitability in chapter 1. Refusing the framing of online pornography as an addictive drug, she traces how infrastructural attachments, networked connections, and sensory pleasures animate self-making projects, attachments, and bodily capacities.

In doing so, we return to the notion of the pharmakon, as it entered cultural theory through Jacques Derrida's work in the 1980s. Pharmakon, the Greek term for drug, poison, and remedy, plays a key role in Plato's *Phaedrus* where Socrates compares the written text to a drug or philter that, promising to function as a mnemonic aid to live memory, breeds forgetting through its dull repetitions (Derrida 1981, 108). Contra internal memory and live speech, externalized writing then entails a homogenization and flattening out of sorts: a similar take on the pharmakon increasingly underpins Bernard Stiegler's (2012; 2013) later work on the technics of memory and attention in networked societies. Derrida (1981, 99) contends that "there is no such thing as a harmless remedy" yet refuses to frame the issue in terms of loss, foregrounding *ambiguity* instead: for him, the pharmakon is simultaneously curative and toxic, partaking of "both good and ill, of the agreeable and the disagreeable." Ambiguous in its overall impact, the pharmakon equally refuses divisions between the "inside and outside, true and false, essence and appearance," the natural and the artificial (103). The notion of the pharmakon helps to frame the problems of technological culture in terms of their possibility for mitigation "through the reorganisation of the tools and techniques of entrapment to create ways out of an impasse" (Moore 2018, 192). Approaching the current intersections of technological, human, and pharmacological bodies through the figure of the pharmakon as a starting point, this book then emphasizes their "*productive* potential," allowing for unexpected transformations and open-ended outcomes (Persson 2004, 46).

Concerns over the impact of technology on our ways of remembering, communicating, and being cut through media theory, from Walter Benjamin's and Siegfried Kracauer's interest in the speeds and rhythms of cinema to Marshall McLuhan's explorations of technologies as extensions of the human sensory system to Walter Ong's Plato-influenced critiques of technology as external, inhuman products eroding both memory and cognition, not to forget more recent techno-pop interventions like Nicholas Carr's *The Shallows: What the Internet Is Doing to Your Brain.* Such concerns have grown ever more pronounced within the current context of data capitalism where much of mundane sociability is organized and monetized through networked means and where the thriving market of digital detoxes, mindfulness, and work efficiency apps aim at aiding focus by removing the external impact of ubiquitous connectivity, promising to restore more authentic and meaningful modes of being in the process (see Syvertsen and Enli 2019). This extenuation of personal connection does not refuse or negate but "is already enfolded in the technological paradigm of connectivity" (Hesselberth 2018, 2007).

Our engagement with critical discourse on pharmakon is also modulated by contemporary encounters with chemical and compu-tational practices, including a basic extension of pharmacological questions to media technologies, as well as the uneven ways these technologies cut across geopolitical zones (and media theory itself). We aim, at once, to move away from familiar divisions between the inner and the outer, human and machine, authenticity and artifice, connectivity and disconnectivity and, at the same time, to shift our attention toward more complex cohabitations where the rhythms and speeds of technology are not merely seen to destroy our em-bodied ways of being in the world but equally afford novel social and political potentialities, experiences, and capacities. As a critical lens, this expanded sense of pharmacology strategically sidesteps deadlocked understandings of technology as either a possibility or a threat in order to aid critical inquiry attuned to the granularities of context. While a limitation of this short book is its orientation toward Euro-American scholarship and practices, it also seeks to examine, and call for more work examining, non-Western and multisited cultures of technopharmacology. Such concerns course throughout the book but are the explicit focus of Ravi Sundaram's contribution, in chapter 2, examining the short video form as a cultural narcotic feeding right-wing populist movements and countermovements in India. Its focus on an emergent biotechnical sensorium pressures existing power relations and changing forms of political mobilization and public affect that are at once locally attuned and globally recognizable.

Addressing this thickening economy of attention and affect, we also seek to reframe discourses of technopharmacological addiction or exuberance, including what Natasha Dow Schüll, in her examination of digital gambling machines, terms *addiction by design* (2012). She traces how gaming interfaces involve tactile interactions and mechanical rhythms that afford access to an affective, cognitive, and somatic "zone" of engaged disengagement with the external world. For Schüll, gamblers are played by the machines that they play with, just as we are played by everyday platforms—be it for the joys of casual gaming, the interest and irritation of TikTok videos, the demands of work, the quests of self-improvement, or the thrill, frustration, and release of porn videos. By interrogating the behavioral psychological underpinnings of machine gambling, Schüll's theorization of the zone as a technique of affective suspension emphasizes a relational understanding of habits or addiction "as a coproduction greater than the sum of the parts" (20). Such work resonates with Wendy Hui Kyong Chun's claim that networked imaginaries "ground and foster habits of using" whose consequence stems from the way they remain unnoticed in our bodies (2016, x). In this way our analyses emphasize not only the material qualities of technology, an influential aspect of current media studies research, but the social and political bodies and practices articulated by emergent technopharmacologies. This relational approach runs through this book, in our engagement with the pharmacological framing of platforms such as Pornhub and TikTok, as well as the technological framing of drugs for enhanced cognition and dreaming.

Media technologies are deployed to the masses as platforms for partitioning time into shrinking audiovisual increments and modulating sexual pleasure across moral boundaries; at the same time, the creative class deploy their own bodies as platforms for biohacking brain states, productivity, and performance. While the pharmacologization of media operates in registers of extraction—of datafied value by big tech—the mediatization of pharmacology operates through regimes of optimization—of cognitive and creative performance by tech workers and urban professionals around the world. Although diverging from meth's destructive links to productivity in alternative drug economies studied by Jason Pine, the mediatization of pharmacology is nonetheless also an attempt to "get more life" (2019, xix). Technopharmacological optimizers get more life by living lucidly while asleep and by living smarter and more mindfully while awake. In both cases, time is of the essence. Yet, as Joseph Reagle argues, the extra life obtained through the systematized living of the hack comes at the cost of breaking the rules for everyone else (2019). Such issues are central to Aleena Chia's contribution, in chapter 3, examining how techniques for rationalizing creativity through dreaming combine rituals of self-optimization with ideologies about the neurological promise of New Age spirituality.

In this way we also depart from familiar debates about pharmakon, turning our attention to actual pharmaceutical technologies, practices, and discourses. Grounded in critical media studies, we trace emergent technopharmacologies across a range of fields, including media and cultural studies, social and political theory, so-called area or global studies, science and technology studies, anthropology, sexuality studies, and the medical and health humanities.[1] What the anthropologist Kaushik Sunder Rajan terms "pharmocracy" is an illuminating example of such intersections. For Rajan, pharmocracy describes the political economy of health shored up by the transnational pharmaceutical industry, which not only exploits economically through pricing, profits, and patents, but shapes basic ideas and experiences of health, value, and democracy (2017, 5). Crucial here is how the performative abstraction of value, as captured by Marxian understandings of labor value, is now expanded to health and to the work of being a body. Joe Dumit terms this abstraction "surplus health" to describe the ways that pharmaceutical companies, in order to maximize prescriptions, have transformed risk itself into a symptom: "risk is now a subjunctive present illness: treated as if diseased" (2012, 16). Such calculative and chemical interventions into bodily capacities, social relationships, and political norms are the focus of Joshua Neves' analysis in chapter four. In the name of optimal or resilient futures, drugs and devices chronically intervene in the present.

The extended time of exception brought forth by the global Covid-19 pandemic during which most of this book was written has brought mundane dependencies on networked media and chemical supports into sharp focus in ways that challenge, and negate, simplified and generalizing diagnoses of social media, internet, and smartphone addiction, as these have abounded in discourses both popular and academic over the past decade. As we are, in many cases, unable to meet up with friends and family, or even to leave the house, mediated communication poses less a threat to sociability than functions as its infrastructural support (Karppi et al. 2021; Paasonen 2021). And as online traffic has soared, so has the volume of user data harvested, stored, analyzed, and sold by data giants, so that the very exchanges that help us feel connected to the world simultaneously fuel an exploitative technopharmacological economy. Combined with the degree to which a return to pre-pandemic routines of everyday life depends on the success of vaccination programs, this particular historical moment makes critiques of both big data and big pharma particularly pressing.

The aims of *Technopharmacology* are nevertheless somewhat different in that, by critically engaging with pharmacological imaginations and discourses concerning bodies, selves, subjects, and actors within neoliberal data capitalisms, we use pharmacology as an analytical lens for understanding datafied and networked lives where human and nonhuman bodies not only relate to but intermesh with one another. Exploring the intersections of technology, pharmacology, and capitalism, this volume asks how both media and drugs participate in the optimization of life within neoliberalism, how they modulate the rhythms, temporalities, and capacities of life on levels both somatic and collective, and how they contribute to both attempts at social governance and the quests for escaping them. Put differently, technopharmacology opens onto questions of platform capitalism that are at once underexplored and urgent.

Our book aims to bring attention to concepts, problems, and texts from adjacent fields focused on pharma cultures and industries— something we only begin to do here—in order both to breathe new air into debates about the platform economy, surveillance capitalism, and the like, and to prepare for new conversations and collaborations regarding our everyday relationships with technology and tonics. *Technopharmacology* contains four chapters that take up distinct encounters between media and drugs, and unfold a larger set of concerns and claims central to the *search for media* to which this book series is dedicated. In chapter 1, "Drugs, Epidemics, and Networked Bodies of Pleasure," Susanna Paasonen examines antipornography discourse framing online pornography as "the new drug" bringing forth a public health crisis. Drawing on and reframing approaches to the pharmakon, Paasonen traces the infrastructures of intimacy animated by networked technologies and the use of drugs and pornography. She contests both normative horizons of the self and prevalent ideas about addiction by foregrounding networks of pleasure. In chapter 2, "The Pharmacologies of Short Video, TikTok, and Beyond," Ravi Sundaram turns to "pharmacology" as a jumping off point to analyze the social media application Tik Tok, among similar platforms. Rather than drug use itself, Sundaram examines smartphone affectivities, everyday forms of augmented intelligence, and the kinetic impact of contemporary "interfaciality" in shaping contentious and public encounters in India.

In chapter 3, "Oneirogenic Innovation in Consciousness Hacking," Aleena Chia examines the pharmacological routinization of creativity by consciousness hackers, self-optimizers who use psychedelic technologies—drugs, wearables, and meditation—to chase altered states of consciousness. Focusing on lucid dreaming pills, Chia explores how spiritual, technical, and pharmacological modes of self-mastery operate through ideologies of neurocentrism— the reduction of semantic content of cognitive processes to neurobiology—an operational premise shared by the behavioral analytic imperative of platform capitalism. Finally, in chapter 4, "The Internet of People and Things," Joshua Neves pushes the Internet of Things into the world of mundane human activity, examining how technopharmacological projects intensify vulnerability and inequality in the name of human enrichment. Paying particular attention to contemporary smartness discourse—from smart drugs to smartphones—Neves examines how the imbrication of big data and big pharma frame emergent tensions between resilience and optimization. Together, the chapters offer a set of distinct but entangled issues for contemporary media theory and join a growing subfield of research at the intersection of the digital humanities and the medical humanities.

## Note

1    The latter is a capacious term describing a wide range of critical and creative work at the intersection of the humanities and medicine (including the anthropology of medicine), science studies, and public health, among others. In addition to other works referenced in the book, this includes: Alaimo 2010, Barad 2007, Benjamin 2013, Bernstein 2019, Connolly 2002, Fuqua 2012, Preciado 2013, Race 2009, Wilson 2015, as well as projects centered on technology, data, and health. A recent special section of the journal *Catalyst* (Dolezal and Oikkonen 2021), examining "Self-Tracking, Embodied Differences, and the Politics and Ethics of Health," is illustrative of the latter.

## References

Alaimo, Stacy. 2010. *Bodily Natures: Science, Environment, and the Material Self.* Bloomington: Indiana University Press.

Agamben, Giorgio. 2020. "Biosecurity and Politics." Trans. D. Alan Dean. Medium. May 13. https://d-dean.medium.com/biosecurity-and-politics-giorgio-agamben -396f9ab3b6f4.

Barad, Karen. 2007. *Meeting the Universe Halfway: Quantum Physics and the Entanglement of Matter and Meaning.* Durham, N.C.: Duke University Press.

Benjamin, Ruha. 2013. *People's Science: Bodies and Rights on the Stem Cell Frontier.* Stanford, Calif.: Stanford University Press.

Bernstein, Anya. 2019. *The Future of Immortality: Remaking Life and Death in Contemporary Russia.* Princeton, N.J.: Princeton University Press.

Berardi, Franco Bifo. 2021. "Freedom and Potency." *E-Flux Journal,* no. 116. https://www.e-flux.com/journal/116/378694/freedom-and-potency/.

Carr, Nicholas. 2010. *The Shallows: What the Internet Is Doing to Your Brain.* New York: W.W. Norton.

Chun, Wendy Hui Kyong. 2016. *Updating to Remain the Same: Habitual New Media.* Cambridge, Mass.: MIT Press.

Connolly, William E. 2002. *Neuropolitics: Thinking, Culture, Speed.* Minneapolis: University of Minnesota Press.

Derrida, Jacques. 1981. *Dissemination.* Trans. Barbara Johnson. London: Athlone Press.

Dolezal, Luna, and Venla Oikkonen. 2021. "Introduction: Self-Tracking, Embodied Differences, and Intersectionality." *Catalyst: Feminism, Theory, Technoscience* 7, no. 1: 1–15.

Dumit, Joseph. 2012. *Drugs for Life: How Pharmaceutical Companies Define Our Health.* Durham, N.C.: Duke University Press.

Fuqua, Joy V. 2012. *Prescription TV: Therapeutic Discourse in the Hospital and at Home.* Durham, N.C.: Duke University Press.

Foucault, Michel. 2004. *Society Must Be Defended: Lectures at the Collège de France, 1975–76.* Ed. Alessandro Fontana and Mauro Bertani. Trans. David Macey. London: Penguin.

Hesselberth, Pepita. 2018. "Discourses on Disconnectivity and the Right to Disconnect." *New Media & Society* 20, no. 5: 1994–2010.

Karppi, Tero, Urs Stäheli, Clara Wieghorst, and Lea Zierott. 2021. *Undoing Networks.* Minneapolis: meson presss and University of Minnesota Press.

Kracauer, Siegfried. 1960. *Theory of Film.* Oxford: Oxford University Press.

McLuhan, Marshall. 1964. *Understanding Media: The Extensions of Man.* New York: McGraw-Hill.

Moore, Gerald. 2018. "The Pharmacology of Addiction." *Parrahesia* 29: 190–211.

Preciado, Paul B. 2013. *Testo-Junkie: Sex, Drugs, and Biopolitics in the Pharmacopornographic Era.* New York: The Feminist Press.

Ong, Walter. 1982. *Orality and Literature: The Technologizing of the Word.* London: Methuen.

Paasonen, Susanna. 2021. *Dependent, Distracted, Bored: Affective Formations in Networked Media.* Cambridge, Mass.: MIT Press.

Persson, Asha. 2004. "Incorporating Pharmakon: HIV, Medicine, and Body Shape Change." *Body & Society* 10, no. 4: 45–67.

Pine, Jason. 2018. *The Alchemy of Meth: A Decomposition.* Minneapolis: University of Minnesota Press.

Race, Kane. 2009. *Pleasure Consuming Medicine: The Queer Politics of Drugs.* Durham, N.C.: Duke University Press.

Rajan, Kaushik Sunder. 2017. *Pharmocracy: Value, Politics, and Medicine in Global*
    *Biomedicine.* Durham, N.C.: Duke University Press.

Reagle Jr, Joseph M. 2019. *Hacking life: Systematized Living and Its Discontents.* Cam-
    bridge, Mass.: MIT Press.

Schüll, Natasha Dow. 2012. *Addiction by Design: Machine Gambling in Vegas.* Princeton,
    N.J.: Princeton University Press.

Stiegler, Bernard. 2012. "Relational Ecology and the Digital *Pharmakon.*" *Culture
    Machine* 13. https://culturemachine.net/wp-content/uploads/2019/01/464-1026
    -1-PB.pdf.

Stiegler, Bernard. 2013. *What Makes Life Worth Living: On Pharmacology.* Trans. Daniel
    Ross. Cambridge: Polity.

Syvertsen, Trine, and Gunn Enli. 2019. "Digital Detox: Media Resistance and the Prom-
    ise of Authenticity." *Convergence* 26, no. 5–6: 1269–83.

Wilson, Elizabeth A. 2015. *Gut Feminism.* Durham, N.C.: Duke University Press.

Vora, Kalindi. 2015. *Life Support: Biocapital and the New History of Outsourced Labor.*
    Durham, N.C.: Duke University Press.

# Drugs, Epidemics, and Networked Bodies of Pleasure

**Susanna Paasonen**

Fight the New Drug is a Utah-based antipornography NGO founded in 2009. Targeting young men in particular, operating in social media, and making use of popular neuroscientific rhetoric, it argues that online pornography is an addictive toxin that rewires users' brains to detrimental effect. This claim is supported by other activist, advocacy, and lobbying groups identifying pornography as a "public health crisis": to date, twenty-nine U.S. states have either proposed or passed resolutions to this effect (Burke and MillerMacPhee 2021). The equation of porn with addictive toxins necessitating yet another "War on Drugs" is further supported by the online community formation around the subreddit NoFap (est. 2011), promoting abstinence from porn use and masturbation (e.g., Burnett 2021; Hartmann 2021; Johanssen 2022; Oeming 2018; Taylor and Jackson 2018).

Pornography is certainly no novelty in the realm of cultural production, nor are initiatives and policies opposing it. The massive circulation of online porn is nevertheless argued to be a qualitatively different beast from sexually explicit content distributed on VHS tape, in magazines, as booklets, and on DVD. As a "new drug," online porn is seen to spread uncontrollably in networked connections and to be more extreme, ubiquitous, and harmful than whatever it is that came before. If porn has been perennially considered toxic in its social impact, then networked media have arguably accelerated its nefarious powers to expansive, epidemic proportions. Porn-addiction discourse, critiqued as a "politically motivated misdirection of public health resources" operating with "a retrograde understanding of both health and media scholarship" (Webber and Sullivan 2018, 192; Ley 2018), comes with a seductive popular pull. Originating in the United States, it has international appeal in reframing antipornography campaigns on biomedical terms as an issue of moral hygiene (Schaler 2000).

The rhetoric of "the new drug" builds on a lengthy tradition of warning against the corrosive impact of bodily practices of pleasure on levels both social and personal. Following Jacques Derrida (1993, 1–2), the notion of drugs is a rhetorical construct rooted in historical context, based on moral and political evaluations, and wrapped up in norms and prohibitions. To label something a drug means positioning it in opposition to both the natural world (as artificial) and social institutions (as a destabilizing, harmful force). As Derrida (1981, 99, 125) points out, *pharmakon,* the Greek term for drugs, signifies both a toxin and a remedy and thus involves fundamental ambiguity of meaning in standing for both a cause and a cure, possibly simultaneously so. Examining the framing of online porn as an addictive "new drug" and broadly making use of the pharmakon as an analytical lens for exploring the boundary work that this entails, this chapter moves from conceptualizations of addiction to infrastructural technological dependencies, connections, and attachments.

In what follows, I work critically through distinctions drawn between the inner and the outer, the organic and the artificial/ technological in discourses of online porn addiction, and propose a framework foregrounding pleasure and excitement as elementary concerns in and for cultural inquiry. Pleasure, as discussed here, is sensory and visceral, frequently framed as a problem in

need of governance and control, yet key to how lives are lived
and attachments formed, and possibly ambiguous in the shapes
it takes.

## Artificial, Addictive Thrills

According to thesaurus definitions, dependence bleeds into addiction when growing in intensity to "the state of being addicted
to something (= unable to stop taking or using it)" (Oxford English
Dictionary). The notion of addiction is used to describe a wide
range of attachments to, investments made, and pleasure taken in
things as diverse as social media, food, music, sex, day spas, work-
outs, and shopping. From the first sex addiction diagnoses of the
1970s and 1980s (Reay, Attwood, and Gooder 2015) to more recent
concerns over smartphone addiction (Panova and Carbonell 2018),
this involves the biopolitical governance of pleasures deemed
socially and morally suspect.

Addiction discourse further connotes a struggle for—or even the
impossibility of—control in the face of abundant and excessive
options (Reith 2019, 2, 62). Gerda Reith (2019, 74) argues that
nineteenth-century notions of addiction were coined in connection with concerns about weakened individual will within liberal
capitalism. The need for ever more intense forms of self-control
then grew in tandem with the intensification of consumption in
deregulated capitalism where insatiable desires met an unlimited
number of consumable objects, "paving the way for an almost
potentially infinite expansion of the field of addiction itself, from
gambling and sugar to smartphones and Facebook" (Reith 2019,
66). Expansive applications of addiction discourse intermesh with
the vernacular of being "hooked" on devices, apps, TV series,
games, and other media objects (Jenkins 2006, 20; Hellman 2009).
Parallel to this positive framing of engaged affective attachment
runs an expansive discourse of risk and pathology where devices
and platforms are seen to enslave their users and diminish their
capacities to act. Diagnoses of internet addiction in particular

have accumulated since the late 1990s in self-help resources and academic analyses alike, and they remain in broad use so that "social media addiction," for example, may simply refer to people regularly checking their feeds (see Andreassen et al. 2012; Griffiths 2012; Reay, Attwood, and Gooder 2015, 9).

As "a kind of streetwise colloquial overstatement" (Coyne 2016, 129), addiction diagnoses can be applied to virtually any activity driven by a quest for pleasure. They function as "shorthand for a wider cultural malaise, expressing a range of relationships with which individuals feel unable to cope" (Reith 2019, 71) and speak of anxieties and moral judgments in neoliberal capitalism (Foddy and Savulescu 2007, 29). Ultimately, the notion of addiction involves the management of pleasures and desires, and judgments on how lives should be lived (Reith 2019, 67). All this leads to an easy conflation of habitual routines with compulsions and pleasure practices with pathological habits.

As the clinical concept of addiction constantly bleeds into broader discussions on pleasure practices deemed problematic on moral grounds (Ley, Prause, and Finn 2014, 96), it is not surprising for it to be a lively trope in connection with pornography, despite there being no uniformity of opinion as to the evidentiary basis of porn addiction diagnoses (Burke and MillerMacPhee 2021; Vörös 2009; Williams, Thomas, and Prior 2020; Reay, Attwood, and Gooder 2015). In the notion of online porn addiction, the compelling powers of networked media meet those of sexually explicit representation, resulting in an affectively charged figure of control lost in the face of miasmic impact.

Framed differently, addiction entails the difficulty of achieving pleasure through objects and substances consumed for the purpose in compulsive manner. Here, addiction involves the pursuit of pleasure that becomes a problem when moving from using a drug for pleasure ("liking" it) to craving it (Ley, Prause, and Finn 2014, 96). When desired enjoyment does not come about, satiation remains out of reach and the addict's life forces are diminished rather

than increased—even if she yearns for more, detrimentally to her
well-being (Bjerg 2008; Weinberg 2002). No longer the master of
her own desires, the addict's autonomy and self-control slip, the
objects of pleasure no longer yielding much joy. While explaining
how attachments to objects and substances become experienced
as a personal problem, this conceptualization separates addictive
substances and well-being, hence bypassing the roles that habitual
drug use can play "in the pursuit and achievement of physical and
mental health and well-being" (Moore et al. 2017, 160). For even
when their consumption is recognized as compulsive, addictive
substances can be engaged with, experienced, and lived with in
strategic ways.

For Eve Kosofsky Sedgwick (1993), the notion of addiction revolves
around the trope of insufficient freedom of will, in that addicts are
seen as driven by external forces beyond their control. As Michel
Foucault (1990, 43) famously argued, the nineteenth century
witnessed a shift from defining "sodomite" as temporarily deviating
from sexual norms to "homosexual" perceived of as a personality
type, identity category, or even a "species" of its own. Sedgwick
suggests that a similar, parallel shift occurred in classifying opium
users as addicts: "In the taxonomic reframing of a drug user as
an addict, what changes are the most basic terms about her.
From a situation of relative homeostatic stability and control, she
is propelled into a narrative of inexorable decline and fatality"
(Sedgwick 1993, 131). This further involved the demonization
of "foreign substances" as the affective, somatic, and cognitive
modulations afforded by drugs in one's degrees of concentration,
alertness, sense of time, or bodily rhythm were framed as corrosive
(130–32). For Sedgwick (133), the notion of addiction involves the
"propaganda of free will" premised on autonomous, self-contained,
and freely choosing subjects. A "user" can be perceived of as a
subject, whereas an addict—unable to choose appropriately or
freely and impacted by powers beyond her control—is something
of an object. Passive and hence to a degree femininized, she dwells
in inappropriate pleasures (cf. Race 2009, 140).

This division between the inner and the outer, Sedgwick's argument goes, builds on a separation between natural and artificial substances and results in distinctions drawn between desires "considered natural, called 'needs,' and those considered artificial, called 'addictions.' Perhaps the reifying classification of certain particular, palpable substances as unnatural in their (artificially stimulating) relation to 'natural' desire *must ultimately throw into question the naturalness of any desire*" (136, emphasis added). As a matter of moral judgment, the boundary work between the natural and the unnatural then revolves around appropriate desires, their subjects and objects, lending diverse addiction discourses a degree of coherence. Addictive substances haunt bodies as perverse supplements of sorts that, in fueling desperately insatiable desires, threaten the moral order of things.

## No, NoFap

Submitting to, and dependent on, external stimuli, the online porn addict is the opposite of a productive, self-governing neoliberal subject. In NoFap's project of self-control and self-improvement through masturbatory abstinence, the porn addict further stands for flawed masculine subjectivity. According to NoFap's Reddit "about community" rationale,

> We host rebooting challenges in which participants ("Fap-stronauts") abstain from pornography and masturbation for a period of time. Whether your goal is casual participation in a monthly challenge as a test of self-control, or whether excessive masturbation or pornography has become a problem in your life and you want to quit for a longer period of time, you will find a supportive community and plenty of resources here.

In his cultural history of masturbation, Thomas Laqueur (2003) maps its transformation from onanism seen as sin within the Judeo-Christian tradition to self-pollution defined as a disease in the late eighteenth century. In both instances, masturbation was seen as unnatural and akin to sodomy as a nonreproductive pleasure practice. As an object of medical intervention and social derision, the masturbator—knowing no moderation—was seen as lost in excessive and unproductive solitary pleasures "with no redeeming social functions" (Laqueur 2003, 232, 235). Such displays of lacking self-control were seen to threaten nothing less than "the basis of civilized humanity" (66). Although concerns over mas-turbation extended to men and women alike (the gender model deployed being binary), there was specific concern over young men wasting their seed, exhausting their life-forces, and turning away from meaningful, productive sociability: onanistic routines were seen to render men dull, weak, nervous, exhausted, effeminate, impotent, insane, and even dead.

In contrast, the 1970s witnessed a redefinition of solitary sex as emancipatory activity resistant to societal governance; "a sign of *self*-governance and *self*-control instead of their collapse" (Laqueur 2003, 277, emphasis in the original). Resorting to nineteenth-century understandings of onanistic self-harm instead, NoFap fore-grounds discipline and individual willpower gained by abandoning porn use, which its community members variously discuss as a bad habit, addiction, and health risk (Burnett 2021; Hartmann 2021). Finished with the fapping, members report improvements in their mental and physical health and masculine vigor. The rhetoric of NoFap casts porn as an artificially stimulating substance threaten-ing bodies from the outside while self-pleasure stands for harmful, unnatural sex. Here, porn and masturbation go hand in hand, just as concerns over onanism emerged soon after the birth of modern pornography (Laqueur 2003, 330, 334; Florêncio 2021).

Following the general template of media effect research, antipor-nography discourses frame porn as an issue of false imagination feeding harmful perceptions of sex and gender. For its part, NoFap—concerned as it is with male freedom and autonomy—comes with a broader aspirational agenda connected to masturba-tory restraint. Whereas antipornography feminism has positioned porn as a symbol of sexual violence against women (as in Robin

Morgan's 1970s extensively recycled slogan, "pornography is the theory, rape is the practice"), NoFap positions young men as the ultimate "unwilling victims of a runaway epidemic" (Webber and Sullivan 2018, 193). The movement's origins have been traced back to a 2011 Reddit post referencing a study by the National Institute of Health claiming that "when men don't masturbate for seven days, their testosterone levels increase by 45.7%" (Love 2013). By mastering their onanist urges, men can then arguably ramp up their masculine hormonal makeup. As no distinction is drawn between the impact of masturbatory and other sexual abstinence on testosterone levels (despite the issue studied being ejaculation frequency), the question becomes that of seed wrongly spilled. Lack of masturbation, the premise goes, makes men more manly.

Journalist Katie Bishop (2019) further explains that "there is also a consensus among many NoFappers (who often brand themselves 'Fapstronauts') that refraining from masturbation can lead to 'superpowers,' ranging from increased energy and confidence to commanding respect from peers or curing social anxiety." Masturbatory abstinence is seen to lead to positive outcomes in the man that one can be—the 863,000-strong Reddit membership being mainly male, although some female NoFappers also place faith in physical and mental reformation. In their discourse analysis of NoFap, Kris Taylor and Sue Jackson (2018) point out that its members frame heterosexual masculinity as innate and part of "the natural order" through evolutionary rhetoric. This involves valorizing "real" sex above the fake in a reverb of broader addiction discourse separating natural desires from unnatural ones. As "dominant seekers of pleasure," these men want to replace dependence with autonomy (Taylor and Jackson 2018, 634). The community formation of NoFap echoes Reith's (2019, 71) point that addict identities are less forced upon unwilling subjects than "actively selected and interpreted by individuals themselves." Within NoFap, addict identities are performed into being by "fostering a (sexual) work ethic, policing one's boundaries, and closing oneself off . . . to better navigate a world that is full of 'unnatural' enticements, such as porn" (Hart- mann 2021, 225).

## Dopamine Overflow

Meanwhile, nineteenth-century understandings of addiction as a "disease of the will" have given way to popularized neuroscience diagnoses of a brain condition (Ley 2018; Fraser et al. 2017). As the brain's pleasure centers are activated when drinking, taking drugs, browsing Facebook, or watching online porn—the argument goes— "synapses and circuits are permanently remodelled by desire and come to require greater amounts of consumption on the same levels of activation in a cycle driven by neurochemical pleasure and reward" (Reith 2019, 64–65). In this take on neuroplasticity, brains become "hijacked" and the addict tied to joyless, compulsive cycles of repetition so that, ultimately, "those who consume pornography more frequently have brains that are less connected, less active, and even smaller in some areas" (Fight the New Drug 2017). Do-pamine is a neurotransmitter connected to expected rewards and key to a range of other bodily and brain functions: as a drug, it is used for treating low blood pressure and circulation. In popular addiction discourses cutting through NoFap and Fight the New Drug, it is narrowly defined as an addictive pleasure chemical, the quest for which impairs users' brains. This line of thought was laid out in Gary Wilson's 2014 book, *Your Brain on Porn: Internet Por-nography and the Emerging Science of Addiction,* according to which porn strengthens certain neural connections over others and, in a vicious circle, hooks men into compulsive routines:

What happens when you drop a male rat into a cage with a receptive female rat? First, you see a frenzy of copula-tion. Then, progressively, the male tires of that particular female. Even if she wants more, he has had enough. How-ever, replace the original female with a fresh one, and the male immediately revives and gallantly struggles to fer-tilize *her.* You can repeat this process with fresh females

until he is completely wiped out. . . . Like that lab rat, you
have a primitive mechanism in your brain urging you to
fertilize the two-dimensional females, males (or whatever)
on your screen. (Wilson, n.d.)

For Wilson, the novelties of online porn result in potentially endless
hormone and neurotransmitter hits feeding a vicious cycle of decline. Similar to "gallant" lab rats inspired by "fresh" females, men
arguably cannot help themselves when faced with an avalanche of
sexual stimulus, as this is how their brains are prewired. Masturbating to porn makes the brain release dopamine and, in altering
the body's biochemical balance, captures it in further pursuit of
pleasure. Recovery is nevertheless possible by "rewiring one's
brain," or that which NoFap calls "rebooting." As with crashing or
otherwise glitchy computers, rebooting is promised to allow for a
clean start.

NoFap is both a peer-support group and a trademark owned
by Alexander Rhodes, long engaged in debate and legal action
against neuroscientist Nicole Prause who has found no evidentiary
basis for porn addiction diagnoses (see Cole 2019). Together with
coauthors, Prause has critiqued the applicability of substance
addiction models to porn use, arguing that variations in sexual
desire should not be pathologized as a disorder simply because
they deviate from social norms (Steele et al. 2013; Prause et al.
2015). Accused by Rhodes of defamation and labeled by the
supporters of NoFap as "a porn and masturbation apologist"
propped up by the porn industry, Prause is part of the scholarly
group "Real Your Brain on Porn" questioning Wilson's addiction
claims. The site for *Your Brain on Porn,* in return, features screen
grabs of Prause's tweets offered as documentation of her de-
faming ways.

This debate on the uses of scientific rhetoric and empirical
evidence follows the long-polarized lines of the U.S. "porn wars,"
waged from the late 1970s to the 1980s and rekindled in the
2000s, the tones of which remain vitriolic (see Duggan and Hunter

1995, 5–6). Furthermore, antagonisms between antipornography advocates and neuroscientists are centrally about the value placed on personal feeling on online platforms. Discord and polarization of opinion is escalated by the confrontational interaction dynamics of Twitter and Reddit, the latter of which Adrienne Massanari (2015) sees as steeped in white, straight, and often misogynistic geek culture in its subreddit community formation, of which NoFap forms a part (on NoFap and the manosphere, see Cole 2019; Hartmann 2021; Johanssen 2022). People experiencing porn use and self-pleasure as negative factors in their lives can find solace and help in addiction diagnoses that seem to speak and offer solutions to the problems they are facing. For a scholar to point out that these lack scientific evidence, then, conflicts with the subjective, felt truth of one's experience. At the same time, David J. Ley (2018, 210) argues that, in pathologizing "otherwise-benign behaviours," serving a profit-driven industry of addiction treatments, and confusing cause and effect, addiction discourse "increases the sense of hopelessness that individuals struggling with their porn use experience." This hopelessness, for Ley, is centrally an issue of shame and anxiety connected to porn use resulting from the pathologization of pleasure practices.

## Infrastructural Attachments

In an interconnected addiction discourse, the constant search for dopamine hits in online exchanges of all kinds is argued to rewire our brains and impair our ability to think, remember, be, and relate (e.g., Carr 2011; Stjernfelt and Lauritzen 2019, 46–58). Through cat videos, winning memes, and endless new updates, the argument goes, online attention economy traps us in its compulsive circuits. The view according to which networked media destructively impair our cognitive, social, and affective capacities has in fact grown somewhat ubiquitous in academia and journalism alike (e.g., Turkle 2011, Lovink 2019; Sundaram in this volume; for an extended discussion, see Paasonen 2021). Accounts of addiction focused on dopamine hits gained from Tinder matches and Instagram likes suggest their frivolousness and banality while ignoring broad mundane infrastructural dependencies on networked media. This, I argue, is ultimately a moralistic move conflating dependencies with addiction and habitual media uses with destructive, compulsive cravings.

If, in contrast, networked connections are understood as infrastructural, and as affording forms of agency within the everyday, the issue becomes one of dependency irreducible to addiction. Following the general tenets of actor-network theory, human agency is dependent on contingent networks composed of diverse actors, many of them nonhuman (Latour 2011), just as the operability of everyday lives is dependent on a range of infrastructural actors from electricity to running water, roads, railways, and network connections. And if individual agency is a distributed enterprise reliant on and constituted by actors that it connects with, relates to, and takes distance from, then the devices and platforms we habitually use are not external objects inasmuch as nodes in networks that constantly make and unmake us. It is not merely the case that we use networked media: rather, these shape our capacities to act (Pienaar et al. 2020, 2). The gravity and depth of our multiple connections to, attachments to, and dependencies on infrastructures means that default separations plying the inner (organic, human) apart from the outer (technological, foreign) fail to hold.

For Lauren Berlant, intimacy signifies "connections that *impact* on people, and on which they depend for living" (2000, 4, emphasis in original). Intimacy, in this sense, is as infrastructural as the networks and attachments that make us (Coleman 2018, 610; Paasonen 2018b). As infrastructures of intimacy, smart devices, and online platforms enable connections and disconnections between people, technologies, bodies of representation, and archives of data. As actors in networks within which selves constantly become, they shape and modulate ways of relating to other bodies in the world, hence being intimate in themselves.

As I have been writing this during lockdowns and social-distancing measures during the Covid-19 pandemic, mundane dependencies on networked media for the maintenance of social relations— along with a range of other connections and obligations—have grown manifest in unprecedented ways. As we are unable to meet up face-to-face and body-to-body, networked connections from direct messaging to video calls have become key to work routines, respites from social isolation, means of connecting and remaining in some kind of touch. Repeating and extending over time, such connections can grow exhausting and frustrating in the detachments and glitches they involve while also allowing for intimacies across spaces that we cannot physically cross or move between.

## Habits

While this particular historical moment is exceptional in the de- grees to which the operability of everyday lives owes to networked connections, these dependencies are also habits gradually formed over time (Coyne 2016, 129–30; Mowlabocus 2016). Wendy Hui Kyong Chun (2016, 1) argues that networked media matter most when they do not seem to matter much at all, namely once they have become ingrained in routines requiring little conscious thought. For Chun, it is not the novel that matters inasmuch as the habitual: repetitions made over time, routines established, and ex- changes continued "without any deliberate pursuit of coherence . . . without any conscious concentration" (Bourdieu 1984, 17, 173). Habits—"mechanical and creative; individual and collective; human and nonhuman; inside and outside; irrational and necessary" (Chun 2016, 6)—involve mundane, embodied attachments that yield dependencies. A smartphone being lost, for example, impacts one's capacity to be in contact with others, find oneself on a map, set an alarm for an early morning wake-up, do payments, figure out a bus schedule, or to distract oneself with casual gaming once on the bus. None of this would have been much of an issue some two decades ago.

Habitual uses of networked media, while being objects of much public concern, are central to our ways of feeling out the world (Richardson 2005). As Jenny Sundén (2018, 69) argues, "The pace of our digital devices blends with the rhythms of our bodies, as a speeding up, or a slowing down, of how our bodies compose with those of others, fostering new rhythms and relations." The inner and the outer, the organic and the technological cannot be neatly told apart from one another since technologies are less foreign substances than intimate, possibly prosthetic things we live with. The question then becomes one of bodily rhythms composed in interactions with devices, apps, platforms, and communication partners that impact our means of acting, caring, remembering, and thinking, possibly in ambiguous ways.

The notion of habit signifies routines but also irritating mannerisms and a craving for drugs, its connotations shifting between the neutral and the negative. This has importance to how the habits of networked media use are perceived. Devices, apps, and sites impact our degrees of focus and our rhythms of perception—as do intoxicating substances used for bringing forth altered bodily experiences (Pienaar et al. 2020). Routines of altering the body's capacity to feel and experience, whether this is done with the aid of online porn, ice-swimming, alcohol, meditation, hormone replace-ments, endurance sports, webcamming, or drug use, become "ingrained in the body as habit, such that they feel deeply visceral and compelling. But they link also to sentient mythologies of taste, performance, affect, mood, and sociability" (Race 2009, 152). Habits formed through repetition become embedded in social norms and practices of social governance that cast some of these as accept-able (a glass of wine after a workday; virtually any form of physical exercise) and others (a bit of ketamine to unwind; a quick session of gangbang porn) less so.

Both drugs and porn can "provide excitement, pleasure, and instant gratification" and "release from stress and escape from boredom. Their effects are transient; their pleasures fleeing, and sometimes habit-forming" (Reith 2019, 84). As instances of experiencing the world differently, such releases add relief, risk, and motion to lives that may feel stuck, or experienced as going around in a predictably dull circle (Cohen and Taylor, 1992, 171, 197). As Kane Race (2009, 166) points out, "Zoning out, getting distracted, losing oneself in something, cutting loose, getting carried away, getting surprised (whether pleasantly or otherwise) are familiar parts of everyday life, and are variously valued." Public concerns on the compulsive, harmful uses of both porn and networked media revolve around escapist quests, the pleasures of which are deemed suspect.

The addictive powers of online porn—"the new drug"—are tied to its habitual uses a discourse concerned with "the control of 'irrational' excess and desire by the rational, civilizing force of society" (Reith 2019, 147; see also Fraser et al. 2017). For Wilson (n.d.), the problem lies in online porn not respecting the division of the inner and outer: "videos replace your imagination, and may shape your sexual tastes, behavior, or trajectory," and as porn "is stored in your brain," it is available on auto-recall "anytime you need a 'hit.'" For those opposed to masturbation fueled by pornographic fodder, technologically mediated practices of self-pleasure speak of inauthenticity that eats away at more meaningful or real ways of sexually relating to and taking pleasure in others.

For Wilson, Fight the New Drug, and NoFap, that which drove nineteenth-century onanists to peril now captures us in compulsive loops of fapping: yet without online porn the authentic self can thrive once again. Their logic is similar to that of digital detox— despite the obvious fact that NoFap operates through networked peer support and is hence incompatible with digital cleanses. Digital detoxes, purges, and fasts are offered as the means of reconnecting with one's authentic self, as well as for crafting more direct and meaningful social connections (Syvertsen and Enli 2020). This involves explicit value judgments drawn between innate authenticity—or "realness" in NoFap discourse—and harmful external actors.

**Keep Safe; Masturbate**

Concerns over online porn comprising a global health crisis are, at the time of this writing, met with an actual global pandemic that harms and kills bodies on a massive scale. When saliva contact presents an active health risk and when the threat of infection looms close if inhaling someone else's breath, public health professionals have heralded masturbation as the safest form of sexual expression—a situation partly, yet only partly, echoing the promotion of safe sex practices within the HIV epidemic (e.g., Race 2018, 13–14, 46–47; Florêncio 2020a). New York City Health Department's Covid-19 sex guidance of June 2020 addressed harm reduction within the pandemic: "*You are your safest sex partner.* Masturbation will not spread COVID-19, especially if you wash your hands (and any sex toys) with soap and water for at least 20 seconds before and after sex." A tip targeted at both frequent users of hook-up apps and sex workers recommended the use of online platforms: "consider taking a break from in-person dates. Video dates, sexting, subscription-based fan platforms, sexy 'Zoom parties' or chat rooms may be options for you" (NYC Health 2020). In a concrete articulation of networked media as an infrastructure of intimacy, public health officials advocate safe, distanced means of sexual connecting.

With the pandemic, online traffic has soared, visits to adult webcam, content subscription, and video aggregator sites included. When the coronavirus was quickly spreading across continents in March 2020, Pornhub reported daily traffic increase up to 24 percent and offered free 30-day Premium membership "to the entire world in an effort to encourage the importance of staying home and practicing social distancing during the COVID-19 pandemic." As "the new drug," online porn is seen to addict and damage users, whereas Pornhub, long attuned to PR opportunities (see Paasonen, Jarrett, and Light 2019, 52–57; Rodeschini 2021), promoted porn as a safe solution, and even as something of a cure, to the discomforts of social distancing.

Networked media and pornography, both together and separately,
operate as a pharmakon across a range of debates while equally
occupying the role of the pharmakos, or scapegoat, accused of
corrupting societal order and hurting well-being (Derrida 1981,
130). Despite the seeming ease of forming a binary between good
(stimulating) and bad (all-too-stimulating, addictive) pharmakon,
such boundary work does not hold as there is much ambiguity
to how networked connections are lived with, and what shapes
pleasures take within them. And if, following Derrida (1981, 103),
the pharmakon disturbs distinctions between "good and evil,
inside and outside, true and false, essence and appearance," then
adopting it as an analytical lens for understanding online pornography means foregrounding ambiguity over generalization and
coining more nuanced understandings of the concerns, passions,
and experiences connected to it.

## The Good, the Bad, and the Exciting

The market of drugs, comprised of licit and illicit drugs and their
uses, illustrates the two-fold nature of the pharmakon: the first
of these markets is ever-expanding and the latter tackled with
diverse "wars" (Race 2009, viii, 7). In the realm of sex and drugs,
the so-called good pharmakon entails function-restoring and
premeditative substances, from Viagra and Cialis to birth control
and preexposure prophylaxis drugs. The realm of the less good
pharmakon, again, involves substances that put bodies at risk by
reducing their capacity to act—as in date-rape drugs—but also
drugs that intensify pleasure and fuel excess, as in recreational
chemsex and slamsex "party and play" drug use (Race 2015; 2018;
Race et al. 2021). Involving "the desire to alter bodily experience,
increase pleasure, enhance intimacy, cement social bonds, and
indulge in erotic practices that may be otherwise uncomfortable or
unthinkable" (Pienaar et al. 2020, 7), chemsex foregrounds sheer
sexual pleasure, contests the notion of organic embodiment, and
alters one's understanding of what the body can do (Hakim 2019,
118; Race 2009, 154).

Writing at the intersection of human bodies, technologies, and drugs, Race (2009; 2018) foregrounds experimentality in how possibilities and preferences are tested out (also Pienaar et al. 2020, 6). Experimentation in intimacy and pleasure, for Race, entail surprises and discoveries as open-ended processes where bodies and their appetites are in constant transformation: "Occasionally something new, unexpected, or queer emerges—a new sensation, an unusual mood, a previously inconceivable way of relating" (Race 2009, 186). Surprises are then key to how the sexual self takes shape through open-ended experimentation: "The most exhilarating pleasures are often those you never imagine could function as a source of enjoyment; that *move* you beyond yourself and make new ways of experiencing yourself and relating to others possible" (Race 2018, 177, emphasis in the original; see also Bollen and McInnes 2006, 112).

Such experimentation can be extended to thinking about sex as playful improvisational practices where pleasure is an end in itself. Through this, bodies learn what they like, what they prefer not to experiment with, and what titillate as future opportunities in possibly ambivalent ways (Paasonen 2018a). Empirical inquiry into porn use has similarly shown it to involve rescues from boredom and experimentation with what bodies can do (e.g., McKee et al. 2008; Barker 2014; Smith, Attwood, and Barker 2015). The scenarios and choreographies of online porn tap into and fuel sexual fantasies and, operating on levels both intensely personal and definitely not, offer vistas of what bodies can do and feel. Sexual experimentation with and without the aid of media make something of a pharmakon in that their pleasures can be tinted in dark and heavy hues, and laced with shame and guilt. Just as the pleasures of drug use can be detrimental to physical well-being, sexual pleasure practices can be destructive in the social attachments they involve, uncomfortable in their execution, highly ambiguous in the thrills they cater, or even the stuff of trauma. Within all this, divisions between the inner and the outer, the personal and the social turn not only porous but impossible to uphold.

According the synopsis of Donald L. Hilton's 2009 book, *He Restoreth My Soul: Understanding and Breaking the Chemical and Spiritual Chains of Pornography Addiction through the Atonement of Jesus Christ,* which combines neuroscientific and theological insight, "Technology has accelerated our fascination with pleasure. Indeed, the power of pleasure has been underestimated." This is undoubtedly the case, even as my understanding of what it means is drastically different. Networked exchanges are centrally about pleasure, the powers of which are indeed both underestimated and undercharted. Pleasure can be rife with affective ambiguity, tinted with disgust, or steeped in boredom while nevertheless remaining key to what drives people's engagements with the world. Pleasure can be plain hedonistic, just as it can be key to social organization striving for political change (Segal 2017; Sundén and Paasonen 2020, 156–57).

For affect theorist Silvan S. Tomkins (2008, 191), "I am, above all, what excites me." If things fail to excite, they simply do not matter—one does not care. As shown by Chia and Neves in this book, some people are excited by the possibilities of increasing their neurocapacity or work performance so that these preoccupations become part of the stuff that makes the self. People can be equally excited by autoerotic sexual thrills even as these are broadly cast as unproductive, wasteful, and hence dubious within the framework of neoliberalism. But if excitement is that which makes the self, then a quest for it is less about addictive desire than about bolstering one's sense of liveliness. Following this line of thought, quests for intensified sensation through online porn and other networked sexual practices speak of the centrality of pleasure and call for acknowledging its importance in cultural inquiry (Race 2009, 187; Florêncio 2020b). Race's (2018, 6) discussion of experimentation extends to scholarly practice as "the need to think and feel otherwise." Such openness, and the ambiguities that it entails, remains crucial in a context where popular addiction discourses cast pleasure as both unproductive and morally suspicious.

NoFap has taken shape in a historical moment where sexual content is, in Stephen Molldrem's (2018) phrasing, *deplatformed* from social media that structure much of mundane sociability. Social media services' content policies and community standards expand the criteria of offensiveness and obscenity beyond the genre of pornography to nudity in artworks, tantric massage photos, and sex education resources. As much of social media frame out not only sexual visual content but sexual communication as inappropriate, sexuality is effectively framed out from the exchanges allowed on these platforms. The 2018 U.S. FOSTA/SESTA (Allow States and Victims to Fight Online Sex Trafficking Act/Stop Enabling Sex Traffickers Act) legislation has contributed to the tightening of social media community standards globally by making platforms responsible for the content that users publish. While arguably aimed at curbing sex trafficking, it effectively impacts all sexual communication and content sharing (See Paasonen, Jarrett, and Light 2019).

This has led to vigilant screening out of offensive "female-presenting" nipples and content that, according to social media market leader Facebook, "facilitates, encourages or coordinates sexual encounters or commercial sexual services between adults." Meanwhile, Facebook has been reluctant to moderate posts inciting political violence in the name of freedom of speech, claiming that this is not appropriate as the company is not a publisher— even as it has been identified as one in the framework of FOSTA/SESTA. This discrepancy in vigilance and moderation speaks of a value hierarchy where sex, broadly construed, is seen as lacking in social value and worth. Even as advances are made in sexual civic rights internationally, sex remains associated with risk, harm, and danger—as in Facebook community standards classifying adult nudity and attempts to hook up as "objectionable content" alongside hate speech and violence (Spišák et al. 2021).

This conforms to a broader logic that David M. Halperin (2017, 3) identifies as "the war on sex": a cumulative effect of many

independent initiatives targeting sex, and especially forms of sex
arousing "disapproval on moral, aesthetic, political, or religious
grounds." Just as sex is zoned out from public urban spaces, the
deplatforming of sex extends cleansing operations to online
platforms in the name of safety and normalcy (Halperin 2017, 6;
Race 2018, 172–73; Oeming 2018). Barry Reay, Nina Attwood, and
Claire Gooder (2015, 7–8) situate the emergence of sex addiction
discourse within the sex wars as expressive of cultural anxieties.
Identifying sex addiction as "a label without explanatory force,"
they argue that its broad appeal owes to vagueness allowing for a
range of actions and engagements to be classified as pathological
(Reay, Attwood and Gooder 2015 105, 163). Building on sex-
addiction diagnoses, the notion of porn addiction is then explicitly
tied to boundary work as a vehicle for "moralistic judgments, the
stigmatization of sexual minorities, and the suppression of certain
sexual expressions and behaviors. The concept of porn addiction is
one mechanism to exert social control over sexuality as expressed
or experienced through modern technological means" (Ley, Prause,
and Finn 2014, 101).

As one extension of the war on sex, battles against porn as the
"new drug" pay no heed to the genre's inner diversity, its ethics
of production, the opacities of the data economy within which it
circulates, or the diverse ways in which people consume porn in
everyday settings. Rather, porn comes across as a bad pharmakon
(and pharmakos) that kills love and intimacy, brings forth erectile
dysfunction, and contributes to rape culture. This discourse
positions porn as threatening the stability and well-being of culture
and society from the outside, just as wars are waged on foreign
lands, or on home fronts to fight off alien invaders. But if porn is
considered the stuff of culture, and sexual fantasies as simultaneously personal and social, idiosyncratic and shared, a war against it
is less of a viable pursuit.

As a heterogeneous realm of cultural production, porn builds on,
plays with, recycles, and remixes cultural tropes, social divisions,
norms, and taboos of all kinds. Like culture in general, it is

polyvocal and diverse, and, resulting from the efforts of amateurs, large commercial studios, and independent kink entrepreneurs, it refuses congealment in any singular aesthetic, political, ethical, or economic principle of operation, even as its circulation is largely centered on video aggregator platforms extracting profits from user data and pirated content. Furthermore, concerns about online porn as a public health crisis have come about in a cultural context where the boundaries of the genre have grown increasingly porous: the war on porn is waged as sexual communication and content flow from diverse sources, often horizontally, and in ways undermining conventional notions of what porn, its products, producers, or markets may be.

The most popular pornographic sites, according to Alexa rankings in August 2021, were both cam sites: Chaturbate (number 47) and LiveJasmin (number 75), with Pornhub at 72, XVideos at 90, and xHamster at 94 among globally ranked sites. Cam sites foreground-ing live interaction sit uncomfortably with common understandings of porn as "sex films" (as used in Prause's studies, for example), as does the success of the content subscription service OnlyFans during the pandemic. Whether it takes the shape of a Zoom-facilitated BDSM session, experimentation with the exotica of online porn, a hot sexting spree with a stranger, or extended messaging with a long-term partner, mediated sexual exchanges are improvisatory activity connected to fantasy, desire, and pleasure. People engaging in such networked sexual play do not necessarily define their practices as pornographic—but possibly as erotic, intense, exciting, and important. The deplatforming of sex involves the weeding out of objects, exchanges, and sources of sexual pleasure that greatly matter as the stuff that excites, and hence also makes, the self.

## Obscure Objects of Desire

Sexual fantasies draw from a broad range of sources—expert advice columns, erotica, things cursorily glanced on a webcam site, classic stacks of Euro Porn, hook-ups reminisced—and are

both open to novelty and tenacious in how they linger. Networked
media, online resources, and a range of cultural products contribute to fantasies and ways of figuring out sexual selves. Meanwhile,
as argued above, diagnoses of porn addiction operate with dichot-
omous distinctions plying the social apart from the technological,
the natural from the artificial, the inner from the outer, the authentic from the inauthentic, the real from the fake, the good from the
bad.

Bearing in mind Sedgwick's (1993, 136) remark on how the pitting
of natural desires against unnatural ones "must ultimately throw
into question the naturalness of any desire," Race (2009, 9) suggests that medical drugs, in arguably supporting "normal health"
(in contrast to drugs altering the body's biochemical balance for
the sheer pleasure of it) reveal both the artifice and the political
stakes involved in the production of so-called normal bodies.
Divisions drawn between normal, supernormal, and abnormal
pleasures evoke the question of normalcy and the governance
of bodies, their capacities and desires, which the figure of the
pharmakon helps to set productively into question. As an analytical
lens, the pharmakon makes it possible to resist, and to refuse,
divisions separating real sex from the apparently fake, good drugs
maintaining innate functions from those opening up novel zones of
sensation, or authentic ways of being in the world from technologically mediated ones.

My argument is for a logic of both/and rather than either/or, where
binary forms of meaning-making are replaced with considerations
of simultaneity, complexity, and ambiguity so that online pornography is seen as volatile and contingent in the sensations and
relations that it gives rise to, and unfixed in its impact on individual
or collective bodies. I further argue for the importance of attending
to the complexity of pleasures and the affective intensities that
they are embedded in. These are key as pleasures and desires in
networked sexual practices are part of what helps bodies thrive,
invests lives with excitement, and expands capacities to feel, relate,
and be.

# References

Andreassen, Cecilie Schou, Torbjørn Torsheim, Geir Scott Brunborg, and Ståle Pallesen. 2012. "Development of Facebook Addiction Scale." *Psychological Reports* 110, no. 2: 501–17.

Barker, Martin. 2014. "The 'Problem' of Sexual Fantasies." *Porn Studies* 1 no. 1–2: 143–60.

Berlant, Lauren. 2000. "Intimacy: A Special Issue." In *Intimacy,* ed. Lauren Berlant, 1–8. Chicago: University of Chicago Press.

Bishop, Katie. 2019. "What's Causing Women to Join the NoFap Movement?" *The Guardian,* September 9, https://www.theguardian.com/lifeandstyle/2019/sep/09/whats-causing-women-to-join-the-nofap-movement.

Bjerg, Ole. 2008. "Drug Addiction and Capitalism: Too Close to the Body." *Body & Society* 14, no. 2: 1–22.

Bollen, Jonathan and David McInnes. 2006. "What Do You Like to Do? Gay Sex and the Politics of Interaffectivity." *Gay & Lesbian Issues and Psychology Review* 2, no. 3: 107–13.

Bourdieu, Pierre. 1984. *Distinction: A Social Critique of the Judgement of Taste.* Trans. Richard Nice. London: Routledge.

Burke, Kelsy, and Alice MillerMacPhee. 2021. "Constructing Pornography Addiction's Harms in Science, News Media, and Politics." *Social Forces* 99, no. 3: 1334–62.

Burnett, Scott. 2021. "The Battle for 'NoFap': Myths, Masculinity, and the Meaning of Masturbation Abstention." *Men and Masculinities,* https://journals.sagepub.com/doi/full/10.1177/1097184X211018256.

Carr, Nicholas. 2011. *The Shallows: What the Internet Is Doing to Our Brains.* New York: Norton.

Chun, Wendy Hui Kyong. 2016. *Updating to Remain the Same: Habitual New Media.* Cambridge, Mass.: MIT Press.

Cohen, Stanley, and Laurie Taylor. 1992. *Escape Attempts: The Theory and Practice of Resistance to Everyday Life.* 2d ed. London: Routledge.

Cole, Samantha. 2019. "NoFap Founder Is Suing a Neuroscientist Who Thinks Masturbating Is Fine." *Vice,* November 13, https://www.vice.com/en_us/article/ywa97m/nofap-founder-suing-a-neuroscientist-no-nut-november.

Coleman, Rebecca. 2018. "Theorizing the Present: Digital Media, Pre-Emergence, and Infra-Structures of Feeling." *Cultural Studies* 32, no 4: 600–622.

Coyne, Richard. 2016. *Mood and Mobility: Navigating the Emotional Spaces of Digital Social Networks.* Cambridge, Mass.: MIT Press.

Derrida, Jacques. 1981. *Dissemination.* Trans. Barbara Johnson. London: The Athlone Press.

Derrida, Jacques. 1993. "The Rhetoric of Drugs: An Interview." Trans. Michael Israel. *Differences* 5, no. 1: 1–25.

Duggan, Lisa, and Nan Hunter. 1995. *Sex Wars: Sexual Dissent and Political Culture.* New York: Routledge.

Fight the New Drug. 2017. "How Porn Changes the Brain." August 17, https://fightthenewdrug.org/how-porn-changes-the-brain/.

Florêncio, João. 2020a. "Writing Theory during a Pandemic." *Identities: Journal for Politics, Gender and Culture* 17, no. 1: 32–34.

Florêncio, João. 2020b. *Bareback Porn, Porous Masculinities, Queer Futures: The Ethics of Becoming-Pig.* London: Routledge.

Florêncio, João. 2021. "Chemsex Cultures: Subcultural Reproduction and Queer Survival." *Sexualities,* https://journals.sagepub.com/doi/full/10.1177/1363460720 986922.

Foddy, Bennett, and Julian Savulesu. 2007. "Addiction Is Not an Affliction: Addictive Desires Are Merely Pleasure-Oriented Desires." *American Journal of Bioethics* 7, no. 1: 29–32.

Foucault, Michel. 1990. *The History of Sexuality, vol. I: An Introduction.* Trans. Robert Hurley. London: Penguin.

Fraser, Suzanne, Kiran Pienaar, Ella Dilkes-Frayne, David Moore, Renata Kokanovic, Carla Treloar, and Adrian Dunlop. 2017. "Addiction Stigma and the Biopolitics of Liberal Modernity: A Qualitative Analysis." *International Journal of Drug Policy* 44:192–201.

Griffiths, Mark D. 2012. "Facebook Addiction: Concerns, Criticism, and Recommenda-tions—A Response to Andreassen and Colleagues." *Psychological Reports* 110, no. 2: 518–20.

Halperin, David M. 2017. "Introduction: The War on Sex." In *The War on Sex,* ed. David M. Halperin and Trevor Hoppe, 1–61. Durham, N.C.: Duke University Press.

Hakim, Jamie. 2019. *Work That Body: Male Bodies in Digital Culture.* Lanham, Md.: Rowman and Littlefield.

Hartmann, Marlene. 2021. "The Totalizing Meritocracy of Heterosex: Subjectivity in NoFap." *Sexualities* 24, no. 3: 409–30.

Hellman, Matilda. 2009. "Designation Practices and Perceptions of Addiction—A Diachronic Analysis of Finnish Press Material from 1968–2006." *Nordic Studies on Alcohol and Drugs* 26, no. 4: 355–72.

Jenkins, Henry. 2006. *Fans, Bloggers, and Gamers: Exploring Participatory Culture.* New York: New York University Press.

Johanssen, Jacob. 2022. *Fantasy, Online Misogyny, and the Manosphere: Male Bodies of Dis/Inhibition.* London: Routledge.

Laqueur, Thomas. 2003. *Solitary Sex: A Cultural History of Masturbation.* New York: Zone Books.

Latour, Bruno. 2011. "Reflections of an Actor-Network Theorist." *International Journal of Communication* 5:796–810.

Ley, David, Nicole Prause, and Peter Finn. 2014. "The Emperor Has No Clothes: A Review of the 'Pornography Addiction' Model." *Current Sex Health Reports* 6, no. 2: 94–105.

Ley, David J. 2018. "The Pseudoscience behind Public Health Crisis Legislation," *Porn Studies* 5, no. 2: 208–12.

Love, Dylan. 2013. "Inside NoFap, the Reddit Community for People Who Want to Be 'Masters of Their Domain.'" *Business Insider Australia.* November 29, https://www.businessinsider.com.au/what-is-nofap-2013-11.

Lovink, Geert. 2019. *Sad by Design: On Platform Nihilism.* London: Pluto Press.

Massanari, Adrienne. 2015. *Participatory Culture, Community, and Play: Learning from Reddit.* New York: Peter Lang.

McKee, Alan, Katherine Albury, and Catharine Lumby. 2008. *The Porn Report.* Melbourne: Melbourne University Press.

Molldrem, Stephen, 2018. "Tumblr's Decision to Deplatform Sex Will Harm Sexually Marginalized People." *Wussy,* December 6, https://www.wussymag.com/all/2018/12/6/tumblrs-decision-to-deplatform-sex-will-harm-sexually-marginalized-people.

Moore, David, Kiran Pienaar, Ella Dilkes-Frayne, and Suzanne Fraser. 2017. "Challenging the Addiction/Health Binary with Assemblage Thinking: An Analysis of Consumer Accounts." *International Journal of Drug Policy* 44:155–63.

Mowlabocus, Sharif. 2016. "The 'Mastery' of the Swipe: Smartphones, Transitional Objects, and Interstitial Time." *First Monday* 21, no. 10, https://firstmonday.org/ojs/index.php/fm/article/view/6950.

NYC Health. 2020. "Safer Sex and COVID-19." June 8, https://www1.nyc.gov/assets/doh/downloads/pdf/imm/covid-sex-guidance.pdf.

Oeming, Madita. 2018. "A New Diagnosis for Old Fears? Pathologizing Porn in Contemporary US Discourse." *Porn Studies* 5, no. 2: 213–16.

Paasonen, Susanna. 2018a. *Many Splendored Things: Thinking Sex and Play.* London: Goldsmiths Press.

Paasonen, Susanna. 2018b. "Infrastructures of Intimacy." In *Mediated Intimacies: Connectivities, Relationalities, and Proximities,* ed. Rikke Andreassen, Michael Nebeling Petersen, Katherine Harrison, and Tobias Raun, 103–16. London: Routledge.

Paasonen, Susanna. 2021. *Dependent, Distracted, Bored: Affective Formations in Networked Media.* Cambridge, Mass.: MIT Press.

Paasonen, Susanna, Kylie Jarrett, and Ben Light. 2019. *NSFW: Sex, Humor, and Risk in Social Media.* Cambridge, Mass.: MIT Press.

Panova, Tayana, and Xavier Carbonell. 2018. "Is Smartphone Addiction Really an Addiction?" *Journal of Behavioral Addictions* 7, no. 2: 252–59.

Pienaar, Kiran, Dean Anthony Murphy, Kane Race, and Toby Lea. 2020. "Drugs as Technologies of the Self: Enhancement and Transformation in LGBTQ Cultures." *International Journal of Drug Policy* 78:102673.

Prause, Nicole, Vaughn R. Steele, Cameron Staley, Dean Sabatinelli, and Greg Hajcak. 2015. "Modulation of Late Positive Potentials by Sexual Images in Problem Users and Controls Inconsistent with 'Porn Addiction.'" *Biological Psychology* 109:192–99.

Race, Kane. 2009. *Pleasure Consuming Medicine: The Queer Politics of Drugs.* Durham, N.C.: Duke University Press.

Race, Kane. 2015. "'Party and Play': Online Hook-Up Devices and the Emergence of PNP Practices among Gay Men." *Sexualities* 18, no. 3: 253–75.

Race, Kane. 2018. *The Gay Science: Intimate Experiments with the Problem of HIV.* New York: Routledge.

Race, Kane, Dean Murphy, Kiran Pienaar, and Toby Lea. 2021. "Injecting as Sexual Practice: Cultural Formations of 'Slamsex.'" *Sexualities,* https://journals.sagepub.com/doi/pdf/10.1177/1363460720986924.

Reay, Barry, Nina Attwood, and Claire Gooder. 2015. *Sex Addiction: A Critical History.* Cambridge: Polity.

Reith, Gerda. 2019. *Addictive Consumption: Capitalism, Modernity, and Excess.* London: Routledge.

Richardson, Ingrid. 2005. "Mobile Technosoma: Some Phenomenological Reflections on Itinerant Media Devices." *Fibreculture* 6, http://six.fibreculturejournal.org/ fcj-032-mobile-technosoma-some-phenomenological-reflections-on-itinerant -media-devices/.

Rodeschini, Silvia. 2021. "New Standards of Respectability in Contemporary Pornography: Pornhub's Corporate Communication." *Porn Studies* 8, no. 1: 76–91.

Schaler, Jeffrey A. 2000. "Moral Hygiene." *Society* 39, no. 4: 63–69.

Sedgwick, Eve Kosofsky. 1993. *Tendencies.* Durham, N.C.: Duke University Press.

Segal, Lynne. 2017. *Radical Happiness: Moment of Collective Joy.* London: Verso Books.

Smith, Clarissa, Feona Attwood, and Martin Barker. 2015. "Figuring the Porn Audience." In *New Views on Pornography: Sexuality, Politics, and the Law,* ed. Lynn Comella and Shira Tarrant, 267–85. Santa Barbara, Calif.: Praeger.

Spišák, Sanna, Tommi Paalanen, Susanna Paasonen, Elina Pirjatanniemi, and Maria Vihlman. 2021. "Social Networking Sites' Gag Order: Commercial Content Moderation's Adverse Implications for Fundamental Sexual Rights and Wellbeing." *Social Media + Society,* https://journals.sagepub.com/doi/full/10.1177/205630512110 24962.

Steele, Vaughn R., Cameron Staley, Timothy Fong, and Nicole Prause. 2013. "Sexual Desire, Not Hypersexuality, Is Related to Neurophysiological Responses Elicited by Sexual Images." *Socioaffective Neuroscience & Psychology* 3, no. 1: 20770.

Stjernfelt, Frederik, and Anne Mette Lauritzen. 2019. *Your Post Has Been Removed: Tech Giants and Freedom of Speech.* New York: Springer Open, https://link.springer .com/book/10.1007/978-3-030-25968-6.

Sundén, Jenny. 2018. "Queer Disconnections: Affect, Break, and Delay in Digital Connectivity." *Transformations* 31, http://www.transformationsjournal.org/wp-content/ uploads/2018/06/Trans31_04_sunden.pdf.

Sundén, Jenny, and Susanna Paasonen. 2020. *Who's Laughing Now? Feminist Tactics in Social Media.* Cambridge, Mass.: MIT Press.

Syvertsen, Trine, and Gunn Enli. 2019. "Digital Detox: Media Resistance and the Promise of Authenticity." *Convergence,* May 16, https://journals.sagepub.com/doi/ abs/10.1177/1354856519847325.

Taylor, Kris, and Sue Jackson. 2018. "'I Want That Power Back': Discourses of Masculinity within an Online Pornography Abstinence Forum." *Sexualities* 21, no. 4: 621–39.

Tomkins, Silvan S. 2008. *Affect Imaginary Consciousness: The Complete Edition.* New York: Springer.

Turkle, Sherry. 2011. *Alone Together: Why We Expect More from Technology and Less from Each Other.* New York: Basic Books.

Vörös, Florian. 2009. "The Invention of Addiction to Pornography." *Sexologies* 18, no. 4: 243–46.

Webber, Valerie, and Rebecca Sullivan. 2018. "Constructing a Crisis: Porn Panics and Public Health." *Porn Studies* 5, no. 2: 192–96.

**28** Weinberg, Darin. 2002. "On the Embodiment of Addiction." *Body & Society* 8, no. 4: 1–19.

Williams, D. J., Jeremy N. Thomas, and Emily E. Prior. 2020. "Are Sex and Porn Addiction Valid Disorders? Adding a Leisure Science Perspective to the Sexological Critique." *Leisure Sciences* 42, no. 3–4: 306–21.

Wilson, Gary. 2014. *Your Brain on Porn: Internet Pornography and the Emerging Science of Addiction.* Margate, UK: Commonwealth Publishing.

Wilson, Gary. n.d. "Start Here: Evolution Has Not Prepared Your Brain for Today's Porn," https://www.yourbrainonporn.com/miscellaneous-resources/start-here -evolution-has-not-prepared-your-brain-for-todays-porn/.

# 2

# The Pharmacologies of Short Video, TikTok, and Beyond

**Ravi Sundaram**

On June 29, 2020, in the midst of an escalating border conflict with China, the Indian government banned the popular short video application TikTok, along with fifty-five other apps originating from China. While TikTok was banned for issues of "data security," the main reason was to placate nationalist sentiments in India's middle classes.[1] Unlike restrictions on cinema and print, where the focus was on specific films or texts, the TikTok ban has been unprecedented in postcolonial history. Two decades ago, in their classic text, Geoffrey Bowker and Susan Leigh Star (2000) argued that infrastructure becomes visible only during its breakdown or absence. Remarkably, India's TikTok ban foregrounded the dependence of the app economy on national sovereignty. The TikTok removal suddenly threw into relief the architecture of a hugely popular platform connecting animated populations and a vastly diverse star system ranging from proletarians to media-industry icons.

Nowhere was this more apparent than in 2020 when video *become the world,* a second moving picture. The vastly varying experiences of work, education, leisure, intimacy, and mourning were suddenly connected by video streams. Ranging from the apocalyptic to the mundane, the multiple ecologies of video suggest a greater ambivalence in the contemporary digital landscape. The exceptional video year of 2020 was a compressed archive of these multiple moods, ranging from the deeply disturbing to tragic, ludic, addicting, and obsessive. Circulating via popular media platforms and phone apps, short videos stitched an evolving, changing event-time, with no clarity on where an "event" begins and ends. Also open to debate are the ways we partition and separate different moods—how do you jump from deeply disturbing videos of terror and catastrophe to a funny meme, or an intimate family forward on WhatsApp? These developments must be seen in the context of a larger distribution of sense (Gabrys 2016), as new milieus emerge when populations interact with media and technical objects worldwide. These new milieus or techno-geographies as Simondon (2017) called them, shape atmospheric infrastructures, which transform the meaning of political affect in the contemporary. Atmospheric infrastructures may suggest a dynamic, turbulent pattern "that is only solid when seen from a distance" (Berlant 2016, 94); equally there is a multiplication of space-times, which periodically draw new populations into media experiences ranging from ambient networks to an everyday screen culture (see McCormack 2017 for a survey).

In this essay I want to focus specifically on the short video, a form shaped by contagious movement and activating different kinds of performance. Short videos are shared across devices, easily compressed, and have a limited time-span. Short videos also demand quick attention. Most powerfully, short video driven by mobile phones have enabled new forms of political mobilization—right-wing populism and its countermovements. Expressed through the app economy, the short video is a political and cultural narcotic in contemporary platform capitalism. It fuels the rhythms of everyday life and produces temporal markers of day and night. The economy of the short video is also uniquely *pharmacological.*

Bernard Stiegler has drawn our attention to the pharmacological condition of technics; a duality that holds both potential and danger, an antidote as well as a poison (1998). Technics (as opposed to technology) allows Stiegler to comment on philosophy, anthropology, and humanity in general.[2] Stiegler pointed to the co-constitution of humans and technics; external mnemo-techniques initiate a grammatization process, which ranges from writing to computer code. A pharmacological condition is both a possibility and an impossibility, since techniques like writing, machine memory, and so on, that allow us to remember (hypomnemata) produce forgetting. Rather than add to a growing bibliography on Stiegler's writings, my interest in this essay is to explore the productive/ restrictive dynamic of a techno-pharmacology in a post Covid-19 era. As Barker (2013) suggests, the "acting-upon" component of Stiegler's pharmacology alludes to an ever-shifting, inventive process, open to ambiguity. I reference Stiegler mainly to explore the possibilities for an expansive model of the pharmacological in a postpandemic world. In the event, I suggest that we need to move beyond some of the legacies of twentieth-century Western critical theory, with its relentless focus on logics of disenchantment, disembodiment, and capture. At the very least, we need to address a changed global media ecology, expanding the pharmacological beyond the Euro-American technogeographies of network culture.[3]

Networked infrastructures create various avenues for collective and micropolitical fantasy. I address this question through an examination of the short-video form. In this context, short videos mark time, fracture experiences, and produce remarkable network experiences. I will begin by framing the short video's history with examples from India, then move on to debates on platforms and the earlier debates on the culture industry by classical critical theory. The final section discusses specific examples of YouTube and TikTok before I close the chapter with a discussion of Stiegler's "new barbarism" and the limiting framework of pharmacology in his later work.

## The Short Video

While video traffic of the recent era seems entirely driven by mobile phone platforms, we need to place this in a longer history stretching back to the beginning of the twenty-first century. There are two elements in the history of the short video that bear mention, as they recur in the post-2010 era in India. In 2001 a news magazine called *Tehelka* publicly released a sensational video of military officers accepting bribes—recorded with a hidden camera. The video made its way to mainstream television and later to multimedia phone circulation. This was followed by a rash of exposé videos produced by journalists and social movements, which quickly made their way into public culture. In the second example, In December 2004, Avnish Bajaj, the chief executive officer (CEO) of Bazee.com, a subsidiary of the U.S. company eBay, was arrested by the Indian police under Section 67 of the Information Technology Act that dealt with the transmission of "obscene" material. The case in question was the sale of a sexually explicit multimedia message involving two Delhi high school students. The clip had first circulated among friends and then rapidly made its way to street media markets and computers of many young men in Indian universities. An Indian Institute of Technology (IIT) student, Ravi Raj, had decided to sell the clip on Bazee.com to a wider network. In the event, not only was Ravi Raj arrested but so was the CEO of Bazee, who was held liable.

Beginning with VHS networks in the 1980s, video radically transformed the postindependence order. In the volatile decades of 1990–2010, video-enabled populations deployed low-cost political technologies, creating new openings for upwardly mobile actors— and sometimes bypassing state and corporate power (Sundaram 2009). The volatility of these decades was mapped onto a dynamic, fast-moving terrain animated by video: public scandals, media stings, pirate landscapes, and an overinformationalized public culture. Hito Steyerl summed up this decade worldwide by drawing attention to a culture of the "poor image" that marked global pirate aesthetics, filled with "countless transfers and reformattings" (2009). The nervous, playful movement of the pirate aesthetic anticipated meme culture of the post-2010 era.

Video's remarkable ecology in India has been documented by new scholarship (Tanvir 2013; Tiwary 2018). Ramon Lobato has written about the centrality of video in cinema's shadow infrastructure worldwide (2012); younger scholars have researched the circulation of media via memory cards and Bluetooth networks in proletarian populations (Mukherjee and Singh 2017; Rashmi 2019). There was an endless, potentializing dynamic that defined the early history of user-produced video in India. The pixelated, shaky videos of this period in India recall the "poor image" aesthetics described by Steyerl. Operating in the edges of the internet economy at the time they were produced, the first generation of short videos moved through a remarkably diverse circulatory engine: Nokia multimedia phones, CDs in neighborhood shops and street markets, pirate sites on the web. The lightly edited, single-shot video of this period is an important legacy, even as it has migrated to more controlled platform architectures in the post-2010 era.

In a notable case in 1991, an Indian court examined the role of video evidence in an important case of public affect involving an excited crowd of students and local police, who resorted to firing their weapons, resulting in the death of a student.[4] The incident was recorded by different handheld cameras, and all the resulting videos were placed in evidence. Video, suggested the court in its final judgment, was preferable to human memory, which was prone to error due to the passage of time.[5] This 1991 case was central in placing video at the center of public affect. As a juridical mode of substituting the human witness, video plays a role in intervening and rearranging the theater of proceedings (Weizman 2014; Schuppli 2020). The framing of witnessing as constitutive of a larger media a priori recalls distinctly Kittlerian themes (Kittler 1999; Siegert 2015). At the same time, the shorter, mobile form of video staged larger debates on the political, of which the judicial forum was surely a constitutive part. The Tehelka sting had cata-lyzed a series of video-driven entrapment events—led variously by informal media players, activists, and sensational media channels. Here public figures, persons of authority, political rivals, corrupt po-licemen would be "entrapped" with hidden video devices recording illegal acts of corruption, police torture, or collusion in antiminority riots. Sting video was an atmospheric infection machine, circulating on television, online portals, personal mobile phones, and finally ending up on YouTube. Brian Larkin's (2013) definition of infrastructures as "conceptually unruly" approximates the volatility introduced by the early editions of the short video; equally important is the relational connections of networks, materials, and media-enabled populations.

## The Political Problem of Short Video

The rise of video significantly disturbed the model of postcolonial power in India, which was framed by techniques of managing public affect. Concerns about media's productivity go back to the colonial management of print. Postcolonial governments operated within a code that functionally separated the social/informational and the media spheres. A censorship board regulated cinema, while central and local government periodically stepped in to stop the circulation of texts seen as potentially disruptive for public order or religious harmony.[6] As William Mazzarella (2013) points out, censorship in India acted as both police and patron, always watchful of carnal excess and a "tipping over" of public affect. The coming of video from the 1990s made the old model unsustainable. The multiplication of low-cost media infrastructures distributed modes of affectivity that proved both attractive and dangerously volatile, eroding the carefully crafted balance of police and patron. With the emergence of media-enabled populations, the older model of a *purely political subject* mediated only by welfare and enumeration became unsustainable.

The government first targeted individual videos for running afoul of censorship or public order regulations. Selective prohibitions on individual media (print, cinema, video) mobilized a performance of sovereignty. Control points multiplied, following the circulatory infrastructure of informal video. Here, control over media circulation was periodically imposed by local police to curate and block

potentially dangerous flows. The speed of the short-video circulation via phones expanded the regulatory targets from individual
media to *infrastructure*.[7] In multiple social disturbances across
India, mobile networks would circulate short videos in a matter of
minutes, proving impossible to regulate under older forms of cen-
tralized media censorship. In recent years government authorities
have used colonial-era rules on street crowds to shut down mobile
connectivity completely in entire districts of the country hit by civil
unrest (Narrain 2017). In the troubled state of Kashmir, mobile
phone connectivity has periodically been shut down for months;
and even when restored, speed has been kept to a minimum, to
throttle short-video circulation.

Beyond the control systems I have described, short video has become routinized in wider transformations. Working in a zone that
variously has been called networked affect (Hillis, Paasonen, and
Petit 2015) or a circulation engine (Sundaram 2015), the short video
has acted as an infrastructure of and relay for different passions.
Ranging from everyday urban encounters, ludic events, and meme
culture, short videos now frame an ever-expansive, atmospheric
infrastructure.

## Platforms, Culture Industry, and More

Designed for a "sensory" infrastructure (Sundaram 2015), smartphone apps are meant to trigger bodily responses: the hand, the
finger, the eye, and the ear. In the early years of the phone this was
dominated by texting, digital photography, and mp3 circulation,
apart from voice calls. With the expansion of smart phones after
2010 the app era has inaugurated an interface-driven aesthetics. As Benjamin Bratton argues, mobile phone apps set up an
"interfaciality" that embeds users in a larger circulation engine.[8]
The app buttons on the phone draw their power from a larger
computational connection, with cloud and data servers elsewhere
in the planet. Writes Bratton, "In connecting one thing to another
by remote control, by action at a distance, the interfacial thing

unfolds out toward the world of other things in looping cybernetic circuits of relay and interruption. It doesn't fold in, it explodes out" (2014, 6). As social movements since 2016 in India quickly realized, editing tools and filters have made video circulation into a memetic engine, far outpacing the early SMS message. The phone interface is now a coveted space, crowded with new applications peddled by companies, government, political parties, and financial technologies. Equally, phone users in India continue to connect with things "nondigital," endlessly photographing paper documents, and scanning images and billboards for memes.

Since 2010 digital platforms have effectively overtaken the legacy of India's chaotic video decades. Beginning with Facebook and YouTube's rapid expansions in the initial years, digital platforms now position themselves as gateways to internet culture for hundreds of millions of new entrants into new media via mobile phones. In India, as in the rest of the world, digital culture has become increasingly identified with platforms, opening up new challenges about framing these shifts within the aesthetic legacies of the 1990–2010 video decades. Platforms are sociotechnical systems that assemble software, advertisers, and circulation channels that aggregate users worldwide. Tarleton Gillespie summarizes the new knowledge logic of a platform as a system that "depends on the proceduralized choices of a machine, designed by human operators to automate some proxy of human judgment or unearth patterns across collected social traces" (2014, 192). As cultural production gets "platformized," a range of creators and users gets drawn into "value" creation, shutting off possibilities of genuine autonomy. As a recent summary put it, platformization "results in the rise of the contingent cultural commodity, which further destabilizes the neat separation between the modalities of production, circulation, and monetization" (Nieborg and Poell 2018, 4282). Platforms are seen to transform cultural production generally, from the integration of cultural industries through software and advertising systems, to the algorithmic curation of visibility of user items, to the collective and "individual" testing of populations in real time by complex and ever-evolving methods of measurement. The trajectory of infra-structuralization (Plantin et al. 2018) suggests models of capture, or dependency, as small producers and artists align their practices for better network visibility.

The argument that the industrialization of culture has debilitating material and psychic effects is not new. The first generation of European critical theory began exploring the synchrony of culture and industrial rhythm. Siegfried Kracauer situated "the masses" in the rhythms of capitalist modernity—expressive of a new sociality and industrial repetition. In Kracauer's *The Mass Ornament* (1995) published in the 1920s, collective expression was aligned with the rhythm of mechanized production. Synchronized forms of collective behavior were presented as akin to mechanized production. This rendered the mass as increasingly functional to capitalist ratio. Theodor Adorno and Max Horkheimer argued, in their chapter on the culture industry chapter in *Dialectic of Enlightenment,* written in exile in 1944, that industrial media played a key role in homogenizing diverse populations into consumers. Broadly, the "culture industry thesis" (as it become known) laid out a map where industrialized mass culture produced docile subjects, framed by false needs that were created by media corporations and serialized production (2002). Variations of the culture industry thesis continued to shape European cultural theory for decades. By the 1960s it was argued that populations were tamed by the postwar boom and mass television. In 1985, Jean Baudrillard published his landmark essay "The Masses: The Implosion of the Social in the Media." Caught in the vortex of permanent (informational) participation, the public was no longer constituted by contingent political speech but absorbed by "transparency."

The video and audio-tape revolutions in the 1980s and the rise of internet culture from the 1990s made the older arguments about the culture industry increasingly tenuous. The platformization thesis has opened a new front in the relationship of technocapitalism to everyday experiences. The informalization of cultural production in the Global South played a major part in destabilizing the hegemonies of the film and music industries in the 1980s and the 1990s. The platform debate often treats informal work as a function of the larger design of contemporary capitalism. As Cunningham and Craig (2019) argue, media "creators" combine precarity with multiple strategies of organization: fighting platform power with online campaigns and alliances with legacy media. In India, small-video creators have sought openings in political movements and have distributed across platforms. Some of these techniques blur platform origins and disrupt oligopolies: much of the video that dominates WhatsApp in India comes from a range of sources: YouTube, Sharechat,[9] Instagram, and diverse political actors and right-wing misinformation channels. While user-produced video remains crucial to platform power, it complicates the relationality of users by expanding the sensory zone: there are leakages, clutter, and multiple attachments.[10]

## Short Video as Opportunity

In 2016, the American networking multinational Cisco excitedly predicted that by 2020, 75 percent of internet traffic in India would be driven by video, largely connected to smartphone ownership (Cisco 2016). This anticipatory excitement has been more than borne out; India remains one of the world's largest consumers of video content, driven significantly by short videos channeled through popular platforms like YouTube and Facebook, which have servers in India. Video also circulated via chat apps like WhatsApp and, until recently, TikTok. India became the world's top consumer of phone-based video in 2020 (Kumar 2020). That was an exceptional year, given lockdowns, social protests, and galloping smartphone usage. This was an overwhelmingly video-driven delirium, beginning with social-movement protest media and memes, followed by Covid19-linked cycles. There was massive Islamophobic video traffic, followed by everyday diaries of the unemployed migrants returning to their villages, and conspiracy theories on a film actor's suicide. In the midst of this was a massive increase in online humor: memes, stand-up clips, jokes of every kind, short video

dance routines by medical workers and hospital staff. We cannot
also ignore the video records of the medical sensorium in 2020:
patient diaries, everyday tragedies, and misinformation videos that
circulated in their millions worldwide.

YouTube's rapid expansion in India in the last decade has made
it one of the main repositories of short video production, along
with popular entertainment.[11] YouTube's combination of formal
and informal practices (Cunningham and Craig 2019) has made it
a remarkably flexible outlet that attracts both the media industry
as well as amateur production (Kumar 2016; Mehta 2020). In India,
YouTube attracts regional language players, content intermedi-
aries, large media companies, fan-based production, informal
producers, and an expanding politically driven video production.
Mash-up aesthetics that proliferate YouTube amateur videos was
first seen by media scholars as an aesthetic reversal. Manovich
(2009) first suggested that with YouTube the political value of
everyday parodic acts held out by Michel de Certeau's (2011) work
was reversed. In YouTube's techniques of bricolage and mix-up,
"the logic of tactics has now become the logic of strategies" geared
towards a media economy (Manovich 2009, 324). This formal
analysis of YouTube came at a time when platform infrastructures were still being rolled out. By 2020 YouTube has been fully
incorporated in the mainstream media economy, with companies
running web series, stand-up comedy, music, and sports. There
are small-scale regional creators, aspirational performers,
small regional media companies highlighting content, hoping to
transition to streaming television. YouTube remains a major venue
of political address in the context of right-wing populism, ranging
from Hindu nationalist rants, alt-right history series, and direct
broadcast of political rallies. A significant component of political
speech on YouTube draws from the direct address videos touching
on contemporary topics by a range of performers: users, regional
and national influencers, vocal artists. Political communication on
YouTube ranges from professionally produced content to amateur
uploads of a single shot, edited quickly on a mobile phone app.

There are regular uploads of violent videos by Hindu right-wing vigilante groups, triggering a chain of connections across other platforms like Twitter. YouTube is a crucial archive as well as a primary source of short video, as longer clips are edited and recirculated on other apps.

YouTube's impact on creators has been studied by a range of scholars (Kumar 2016). Others have focused on how the idea of region becomes significant in YouTube's trajectory of localization (Mohan and Punathambekar 2019). YouTube remains the most visible example of platformization: with proliferating value chains of advertisers, producers, curation systems, and adaptive algorithmic models. In the context of a multilingual, informalized network of cultural production space like India, YouTube remains distinctive in its spatial ambition. Unless subject to takedown notices by courts or pressures from the regime, YouTube has successfully incorporated a reasonable selection of the underground and edge zones of early video culture that can be sourced in multiple versions on the platform. In recent years, YouTube remains a crucial repository for social-movement videos,[12] minority fan cultures, violent trophy videos of Hindu nationalist vigilantes. In every sense YouTube's gateway function has been reinforced—this being a function as well as structural design of platform power.

Finally, perhaps more than ever before, YouTube is the site of an inventive pharmacology. The case of Munawar Faruqui, a popular young Muslim YouTube comic in India is a good example.[13] Muslim comics face a fraught existence on YouTube in India, always under threat from an Islamophobic Hindu nationalist regime and criticism from the larger Muslim community. For young Muslim performers in India, YouTube and other spaces in the platform industry is a rapidly shrinking terrain where they can be heard and earn a living. On January 1, 2021, Faruqui was arrested in a club in Indore, central India, on the complaint of Hindu nationalist vigilante groups for "offending religious sentiment" in his performance, drawing a charge under Section 295 of the colonial-era penal code. Short video clips of other satirical performances were provided as evidence by the vigilantes—none mention a religion nor were

they from the club's performance (Purohit 2021). Here we can see
the anthropology of media via an Indian lens: a global platform;
informal cultural producers hoping to reenchant the world; the
toxic combinations of Hindu nationalism, police law, and the working out of political affect. Equally at play here is an always shifting
geography of affect: users access media in multiple formats and
platforms, cultivating relations of dependence and indifference.[14]
There is a tipping over of scales and moods: larger video events
scatter into smaller encounters, microatmospheres that offer
multiple entry and exit points.

## The TikTok Phenomenon

The short frenetic period of TikTok's operations in India recalled
the storms that the early years of analog video generated. TikTok
produced animated bodies and strange disturbances unseen
in India (Figure 2.1). Even the staid governmental machine was
infected by TikTok: there were videos of police dancing in jails,[15]
doctors and health workers swinging to music before surgical
procedures, and paramilitary forces performing masculinist com-
mando salutes before illegal encounters. The banning of TikTok
threw light on a whole generation of subaltern performers who
had rapidly emerged with the expansion of low-cost mobile phones
and cheap mobile data.[16] Spread across India's small towns and
rural areas, TikTok artists included agricultural workers, farmers,
urban migrants, women and men, street cooks, LGBTQ performers.
Recalling the turbulent history of early video in India, TikTok artists
recorded their performance in a makeshift architecture—often
with borrowed mobile phones. Not unlike early video, there was
a churning of the class and spatial order, as vast numbers of
rural and urban proletarians entered the force of the informal
and ephemeral category of "creators." In every sense there was
a radicalization of the outward expressivity that mobile phones
promised. Suraj Chavan, a proletarian TikTok "star" from a village
in Western Maharashtra (Figure 2.2) made his money not just from
the app but from local networks of sponsors and regional support
structures (Goyal 2020).

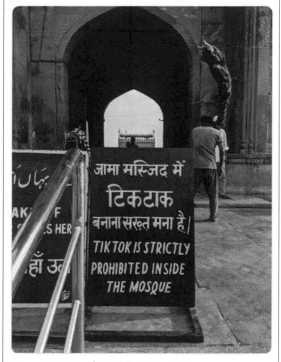

[Figure 2.1]. TikTok shaped the contests of public culture in India, which were referenced in many social media platforms. This Twitter comment on a prohibition notice outside Delhi's main mosque is a good example.

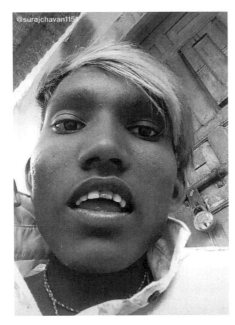

[Figure 2.2]. Suraj Chavan, rural TikTok performer from Western India.

There were village performers, migrant workers, and a whole new generation of working-class women who began making their presence felt in TikTok's universe. A good example is a former TikTok star, Arti—a woman worker from North India (Figure 2.3). Arti toiled in the day and produced her videos at night. The videos show a remarkable combustible dynamic, a controlled body movement, syncing to a popular Hindi song.

Initiated by a Chinese company Bytedance, TikTok began in 2014, from an app called Music.ly. In recent years TikTok has become the single most downloaded application in many countries of the world. Until it was banned by the Indian government, TikTok was estimated to have been downloaded 500 million times in India. TikTok was innovative in its use of a differential video speed. There was a fifteen-second limit to the video, while a range of augmented-reality interfaces (AR) helped enhance the shortened

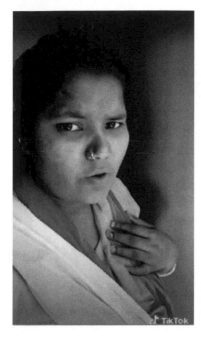

[Figure 2.3]. Arti, TikTok
working-class performer,
@revatil

length. TikTok transformed the experience of video into a playful,
kinetic drive, mixing animation and speed, activating parts of the
body, and triggering spatial expansion and contraction. There is a
special focus on bodily and nervous energy, all geared to kinetic
movement in connective environments. TikTok is emblematic of
the postcinematic move described by Shaviro, where cameras are
now the "*machines for generating affect,* and for capitalizing upon,
or extracting value from, this affect" (2010, 3; emphasis in original).
The financialization of the moving body is linked to a temporal
cycle (TikTok's motto is "make every second count"). As I have
pointed out, TikTok's motion techniques combine AR filters, but in
the Indian case lip-sync techniques proved particularly powerful.
TikTok's "challenges" have mobilized the larger corpus of film culture, notably the productive use of the gestural (Chakravarty 2019.)
The app mobilizes every media innovation of twentieth-century

technics: different speed of the frame and a bodily enervation that extends to the athletic. We have animation, the computational turn, and video game history. The recommendation engine of TikTok uses a familiar model of personalization, but the fifteen-second clip blurs and mobilizes different kinds of performativity, ranging from the comic to the aggressive.

TikTok has a monetization engine that draws from models of online gift giving developed in China, exemplifying a wider landscape of what Shaviro calls an overfinancialized, accelerationist aesthetics. This is the materialization of real subsumption, where the value form spreads to all forms of life.[17] TikTok also uses gamification techniques to stimulate and retain user interest. Gamified design creates levels of users and stars through the accumulation of hearts and diamonds, through an emerging influencer network that is often locally embedded. Gamification is a central component of optimization in new media (Zhang, Xiang, and Hao 2019) and crucial to the way TikTok's algorithm predicts and manages users. Its algorithm promotes instant connections with intuition, where augmented intelligence intervenes and reformats affective environments. Benjamin Bratton (2014) calls this the aggressive subtitling of the world through the AR functions of app interfaces. Since TikTok is embedded in a socially diverse circulation engine, it draws the edges of platform culture. These edge zones include networks of violence, subaltern stardom, and minority political cultures (Ramesh n.d.). Following a court order, in India alone TikTok removed 8 million videos in 2019, the application has also been referenced in caste wars and right-wing mobilization (Jalan 2019).

This combination of postcinematic design and platformization is not the only feature of TikTok's success. The mobilization of bodies-in-motion in homes, public offices, and jails may suggest fully mediatic bodies geared to an attention economy. Equally, the tipping over of bodily action also recalls older investments of twentieth-century critical theory with play and innervation. The late Miriam Hansen (2004) wrote about Walter Benjamin's "gamble" with technology, where utopian possibilities of play and "innervation" were released by new technologies through "mixing," thus exceeding its original capitalist purpose. Benjamin was particularly fascinated by Chaplin's movements. Benjamin wrote:

> The innovation of Chaplin's gestures is that he dissects the expressive movements of human beings into a series of minute innervations. Each single movement he makes is composed of a succession of staccato bits of movement. Whether it is his walk, the way he handles his cane, or the way he raises his hat—always the same jerky sequence of tiny movements applies the law of the cinematic image sequence to human motorial functions. (2003, 94)

Early motion capture from the chronophotographic experiments of Étienne-Jules Marey and Eadweard Muybridge all the way up to the direct address of the cinema of attractions foregrounded technologized, ambulatory bodies. The possibility of innervation as contagious movement, the "gamble" with technology that Benjamin dreamed of, has been fully realized in TikTok's model of acceleration. Despite, or in spite of, its cheerful overcommodified fervor, TikTok generated various meters of affect: play, laughter, and violence. Here application design and optimized populations collide with other objects and spaces, producing unintended public events. What we see are different microtemporalities of affect: play, horror, laughter, and addictive return.

## From Culture Industry to a New "Barbarism"

Shortly before his unexpected passing, Bernard Stiegler published the *Age of Disruption: Technology and Madness in Computational Capitalism* (2019). The book is Stiegler's horrified reflection on what he saw as the new "barbarism" that emerged from a constellation of Big Data, terror attacks, and computational capitalism. Stiegler was significantly referencing Horkheimer and Adorno's *Dialectic of Enlightenment,* and in particular, the chapter on the culture industry. For Stiegler, the new kind of barbarism was a fulfillment

of the prediction of the *Dialectic of Enlightenment* in far more radical circumstances, defined by an "algorithmic governmentality."
What had changed, says Stiegler, "is the systematic exploitation
and physical reticulation of interindividual and transindividual
relations—serving what is referred to today as the 'data economy,'
itself based on data-intensive computing, or 'big data,' which has
been presented as the 'end of theory'" (Steigler 2019, 7). While
Stiegler had earlier called attention to the pharmacological nature
of Marx's theory of proletarianization, the reference to *Dialectic of
Enlightenment* marked his increasing distress with developments in
platform capitalism.

It is widely recognized that Adorno and Horkheimer followed and
transcended the initial impulse of the Weberian-Marxist tradition laid by Lukacs's *History and Class Consciousness* (1972). The
*Dialectic of Enlightenment* was the *Communist Manifesto* in reverse,
overturning the optimistic modernism of Marx's text. Adorno and
Horkheimer combined a critical counter-Enlightenment with an
analysis of the culture industry. The aesthetic of disenchantment
so central to the Frankfurt School is fully rearticulated by Stiegler in
the age of disruption:

> Digital reticulation penetrates, invades, parasitizes, and
> ultimately destroys social relations at lightning speed,
> and, in so doing, neutralizes and annihilates them from
> within, by outstripping, overtaking, and engulfing them.
> Systemically exploiting the network effect, this *automatic
> nihilism* sterilizes and destroys local culture and social life
> like a neutron bomb: what it dis-integrates, it exploits,
> not only local equipment, infrastructure, and heritage,
> abstracted from their socio-political regions and enlisted
> into the business models of the Big Four, but also psy-
> chosocial energies—both of individuals and of groups—
> which, however, are thereby depleted. (2019, 7)

For Stiegler, in the contemporary "hyperindustrial" era, digital
technologies produce a loss of individuation, addiction, and a

"symbolic misery" (2010). While Stiegler called for a reenchantment of the word with the aid of technics, even some of his earlier concerns echo those of the Frankfurt School in the 1940s: the culture industry and the rationalization/grammatization process, the displacement of memory, and the generation of false needs.[18] The return of the themes of classical critical theory is no surprise given the context of apocalyptic post-Anthropocene thought and the hegemony of computational capitalism. The progressive reduction of sources of critique haunted classical critical theory, a platform-dominated apocalyptic thinking seems to pervade contemporary Western avant-garde cultural theory (Paasonen 2020). As twentieth-century cultural and media theory struggled with notions of disenchantment and externalized erosions of subjectivity, it is more than urgent that in a postpandemic context we move to an ecologically aware notion of media. Here pharmacology becomes expansive rather than binary, a mode of attending to multiple points of departure. As I suggest in this essay, even platform-based short videos suggest a more ambiguous story. There are continuing connections with earlier, analog infrastructures. Even in the context of a rising platform capitalism and aggressive right-wing populism, we witness sites of micropolitical action, minor intimacies, and new mobilities. These different scales of intensity and situational encounters sit uneasily with the model of a hegemonic platform economy lulling media-addicted populations into distraction or consensus. This is not to deny the import of Stiegler's agonized questions about the state of the world in his *Age of Disruption* but to propel them into new points of departure. While many of twentieth-century media theorists' brilliant insights will surely remain relevant, we may need to update our media theories for a different epoch after the pandemic.

## Notes

1 "Explained: How Ban of TikTok and Other Chinese Apps Will Be Enforced; the Impact for Indian Users." *The Indian Express* (blog), July 4, 2020, https://indian express.com/article/explained/india-bans-chinese-apps-impact-explained -6482150/.

2   Stiegler's ideas of technics and pharmacology critically engage with the Heideg-
    gerian notion of *tekhnē* and Derrida's pharmakon.

3   The Lisbon earthquake of 1755 is widely acknowledged to have shaken intellec-
    tual life in Europe, after which scientific and secular explanations came to the
    fore. It remains to be seen how the intellectual implications of the pandemic
    will play out. Given the way network culture has been central to the shaping of
    the pandemic, a long overdue reckoning with the legacies of Western media
    and cultural theory might emerge.

4   *P. V. Kapoor and Anr. v. Union of India and Anr.* on September 6, 1991.

5   "Such witnesses may not tell the whole truth, intentionally or unintentionally,
    specially[*sic*] in view of the fact that the testimony would be recorded long
    after the events have taken place. With the passage of time, the memory of the
    witness may become blurred." *P. V. Kapoor and Anr. v. Union of India and Anr.* on
    September 6, 1991.

6   What Michal Warner (2002) has called media's "fruitful perversity" was asso-
    ciated in India's twentieth-century history with potential public disturbance.
    Here the circulation of transgressive media forms was tied to dangerous public
    affect and excitable crowds. This brought about radical changes in the Indian
    constitution tied to speech-based offences, many of which would play out in
    the video and the contemporary era. In the postindependence period, "public
    order" was added as an exception to free speech under Article 19, with the first
    amendment to the Indian Constitution. In addition, there are speech-restrictive
    laws such as Sections 153A and 295A of the Indian Penal Code (IPC). Section
    153A of the IPC criminalizes the promotion of enmity between groups of peo-
    ple on grounds such as religion and race. Section 295A of the IPC criminalizes
    the deliberate and malicious outraging of religious feelings of any class by
    insulting its religion or religious beliefs. All these articles have been deployed in
    the last two decades when dealing with mobile video.

7   There are more than a billion mobile phones in India today. Close to 700
    million have broadband/data access (Telecom Regulatory Authority of India
    2020). For closures of infrastructure, section 144 of the Indian Penal Code (IPC)
    originally for crowd control has been used.

8   Machine intelligence as a transformative or parallel force in human action is
    referenced in public debates in India on politics, environment, privacy. Public
    debates on data privacy, Facebook/Cambridge Analytica, the use of bots in
    politics, and sensors for recording environmental data are widespread in India
    as elsewhere in the world. The references to the technological and political
    axis of augmentation (Pasquinelli 2015) is not a just a theoretical question, the
    landmark Indian Supreme Court Right judgment affirming the right to privacy
    had a long section on data and machine action. Supreme Court of India Justice,
    *K. S. Puttaswamy (Retd) . . . v. Union of India and Ors.* On 24 August, 2017, https://
    indiankanoon.org/doc/91938676/.

9   Sharechat is a popular app for Indian language users.

10  We must also not forget the role of national states that may periodically re-
    strict and renegotiate platform power. Apart from the TikTok ban, the Indian

government has pushed back against Twitter. Users may also periodically deploy strategies of exit: millions in the Global South sought refuge in Signal and Telegram when WhatsApp changed its privacy settings in 2020. "WhatsApp Delays Privacy Changes Amid User Backlash," *New York Times,* January 15, 2021, https://www.nytimes.com/2021/01/15/technology/whatsapp-privacy-changes -delayed.html.

11   Useful for my own research, the archive of former TikTok video stars has migrated to YouTube. All political videos as well as many popular memes make it to YouTube.

12   In tragic reversals of publicity, police have used videos once shared on phones uploaded on YouTube to prosecute social movement activists.

13   "Munawar Faruqui—YouTube," https://www.youtube.com/channel/UC4aTcVT ewbHtLeV8eK3enwA. Accessed January 18, 2021.

14   Faruqui's videos were viewed on YouTube, PIP(picture in picture) windows in WhatsApp and Sharechat (an Indian app), and mashed up on Islamophobic Telegram channels.

15   See https://youtu.be/d-PbuIlhOOs?t=7.

16   Sanatan Kumar Mahto and his elder sister Savitri Kumari, TikTok performers from rural India, told *The Wire,* "This is a platform of the marginalized, people from rural India and those who don't come from rich families" (Srivastava 2020).

17   Shaviro (2015) suggests that accelerationism is ineffective as a political strategy, even while it shows promise as an aesthetic one. Aesthetic accelerationism is posttransgressive, in that it is defined by an aesthetic *inefficacy*. Under the logic of late capitalism, transgression has been fully incorporated as a successful model of market optimization.

18   For a discussion of Stiegler's relationship to Adorno and Horkheimer's notion of the culture industry see Crogan 2013.

## References

Barker, Stephen. 2013. "Techno-Pharmaco-Genealogy." In *Stiegler and Technics,* ed. Christina Howells and Gerald Moore, 259–75. Edinburgh: Edinburgh University Press.

Baudrillard, Jean. 1985. "The Masses: The Implosion of the Social in the Media." Trans. Marie Maclean. *New Literary History* 16, no. 3: 577–89. https://doi.org/10.2307 /468841.

Benjamin, Walter. 2003. *Walter Benjamin: Selected Writings, Volume 3, 1935–1938.* Trans. Edmund Jephcott et al., ed. Howard Eiland and Michael W. Jennings. Cambridge, Mass.: Harvard University Press.

Berlant, Lauren. 2016. "The Commons: Infrastructures for Troubling Times." *Environment.* MISSING PART OF BIB ENTRY.

Bowker, Geoffrey C., and Susan Leigh Star. 2000. *Sorting Things Out: Classification and Its Consequences.* Cambridge, Mass.: MIT Press.

Bratton, Benjamin H. 2014. "On Apps and Elementary Forms of Interfacial Life: Object, Image, Superimposition." In *The Imaginary App,* ed. Paul D. Miller and Svitlana Matviyenko 3–16. Cambridge, Mass.: MIT Press, 2014.

Chakravarty, Amrita. 2019. *Expanding the Archive: Reiterations of Film(i) History in Contemporary Media, Art, and Cinema.* M.Phil., Delhi: Jawaharlal Nehru University.

Cisco. 2016. "India 2020 Forecast Highlights." VNI Complete Forecast Highlights.

Crogan, Patrick, 2013. "Experience of the Industrial Temporal Object." In *Stiegler and Technics.* Ed. Christina Howells, and Gerald Moore, 102–18. Edinburgh: Edinburgh University Press.

Cunningham, Stuart, and David Craig. 2019. "Creator Governance in Social Media Entertainment." *Social Media+ Society* 5, no. 4: 1–11.

De Certeau, Michel. 2011. *The Practice of Everyday Life.* 3d ed. Berkeley, Calif.: University of California Press.

Gabrys, Jennifer. 2016. *Program Earth: Environmental Sensing Technology and the Making of a Computational Planet.* Minneapolis: University of Minnesota Press.

Gillespie, Tarleton. 2014. "The Relevance of Algorithms." In *Media Technologies: Essays on Communication, Materiality, and Society,* Ed. Tarleton Gillespie, Pablo J. Boczkowski, and Kirsten A. Foot, 167–93. Cambridge, Mass.: The MIT Press.

Goyal, Prateek. 2020. "This Daily Wager Turned TikTok Star Learned to Monetise His Videos. Three Weeks Later, the App Was Banned." *Newslaundry.* July. https://www.newslaundry.com/2020/07/04/this-daily-wager-turned-tiktok-star-learned-to-monetise-his-videos-three-weeks-later-the-app-was-banned. Accessed September 27, 2020.

Hansen, Miriam Bratu. 2004. "Room-for-Play: Benjamin's Gamble with Cinema." *October109*:3–45. http://www.jstor.org/stable/3397658.

Hillis, Ken, Susanna Paasonen, and Michael Petit. 2015. *Networked Affect.* Cambridge, Mass.: MIT Press.

Horkheimer, Max, and Theodor W. Adorno. 2002. *Dialectic of Enlightenment.* Trans. Gunzelin Noeri. Stanford, Calif.: Stanford University Press.

Jain, Aashika. n.d. "TikTok Banned in India: How Social Media Influencers Are Protecting Their Finances." *Forbes.* https://www.forbes.com/sites/advisorindia/2020/07/01/tiktok-banned-in-india-how-social-media-influencers-are-protecting-their-finances/. Accessed September 24, 2020.

Jalan, Trisha. 2019. "Madras HC May Hold TikTok in Contempt If It Fails to Moderate 'Negative,' 'Inappropriate,' or 'Obscene' Content." *MediaNama* (blog). May 6, 2019. https://www.medianama.com/2019/05/223-madras-hc-tiktok-order/. Accessed September 27, 2020.

Kittler, Friedrich A. 1999. *Gramophone, Film, Typewriter.* Stanford, Calif.: Stanford University Press.

Kracauer, Siegfried. 1995. *The Mass Ornament: Weimar Essays.* Cambridge, Mass.: Harvard University Press.

Kumar, Chitranjan. 2020. "Indians Watch over 5 Hours of Online Video Content per Day, Most in the World: Survey." *Business Today.* June 24, 2020. https://www.businesstoday.in/latest/trends/indian-viewers-consume-the-most-online-video-content-per-day-survey/story/407904.html. Accessed September 28, 2020.

Kumar, Sangeet. 2016. "Online Entertainment| YouTube Nation: Precarity and Agency in India's Online Video Scene. " *International Journal of Communication* 10: 5608–25.

Larkin, Brian. 2013. "The Politics and Poetics of Infrastructure. " Annual Review of Anthropology 42 (1): 327–43. https://doi.org/10.1146/annurev-anthro-092412 -155522.

Li, Han. 2020. "From Disenchantment to Reenchantment: Rural Microcelebrities, Short Video, and the Spectacle-ization of the Rural Lifescape on Chinese Social Media." *International Journal of Communication* 14: 3769–88

Lobato, Ramon. 2012. *Shadow Economies of Cinema: Mapping Informal Film Distribution.* London: British Film Institute.

Lukács, Georg. 1972. *History and Class Consciousness: Studies in Marxist Dialectics.* Trans. Rodney Livingstone. Cambridge, Mass.: The MIT Press.

Manovich, Lev. 2009. "The Practice of Everyday (Media) Life: From Mass Consumption to Mass Cultural Production?" *Critical Inquiry* 35, no. 2: 319–31.

Mazzarella, William. 2013. *Censorium: Cinema and the Open Edge of Mass Publicity.* Durham, N.C.: Duke University Press.

McCormack, Derek P. 2017. "Elemental Infrastructures for Atmospheric Media: On Stratospheric Variations, Value and the Commons." *Environment and Planning D: Society and Space* 35, no. 3: 418–37.

Mehta, Smith. 2020. "Localization, Diversification, and Heterogeneity: Understanding the Linguistic and Cultural Logics of Indian New Media." *International Journal of Cultural Studies* 23, no. 1: 102–20.

Mehta, Smith, and D. Bondy Valdovinos Kaye. 2019. "Pushing the Next Level: Investigating Digital Content Creation in India." *Television & New Media.* https://doi.org /10.1177/1527476419861698.

Mohan, Sriram, and Aswin Punathambekar. 2019. "Localizing YouTube: Language, Cultural Regions, and Digital Platforms." *International Journal of Cultural Studies* 22, no. 3: 317–33. https://doi.org/10.1177/1367877918794681.

Mukherjee, Rahul, and Abhigyan Singh. 2017. "MicroSD-Ing 'Mewati Videos': Circulation and Regulation of a Subaltern-Popular Media Culture." In *Asian Video Cultures: In the Penumbra of the Global.* Ed. Joshua Neves and Bhaskar Sarkar, 133–57. Durham, N.C.: Duke University Press.

Narrain, Siddharth. 2017. "Dangerous Speech in Real Time: Social Media, Policing, and Communal Violence." *Economic and Political Weekly* 52 , no. 34. https://www .epw.in/engage/article/dangerous-speech-real-time-social-media-policing-and -communal-violence.

Nieborg, David B., and Thomas Poell. 2018. "The Platformization of Cultural Production: Theorizing the Contingent Cultural Commodity." *New Media & Society* 20, no. 11: 4275–92.

Paasonen, Susanna. 2020. "Distracted Present, Golden Past?" *Media Theory* 4, no. 2: 11–32.

Pasquinelli, Matteo, ed. 2015. *Alleys of Your Mind: Augmented Intelligence and Its Traumas.* Leuphana: meson press.

Plantin, Jean-Christophe, Carl Lagoze, Paul N. Edwards, and Christian Sandvig. 2018.

"Infrastructure Studies Meet Platform Studies in the Age of Google and Facebook." *New Media & Society* 20, no. 1: 293–310.

Purohit, Kunal. 2021. "Muslim Comic Did Not Joke about Hindus, But 'It Doesn't Matter': Police Chief." *Article 14*. January 14. https://www.article-14.com/post/muslim-comic-did-not-joke-about-hindus-but-it-doesn-t-matter-police-chief. Accessed February 2, 2021.

Ramesh, Zijah Sherwani, Mythreyee. n.d. "'TikTok Shared Queer Happiness & Sorrow': LGBTQ Members on App Ban." *The Quint*. https://www.thequint.com/neon/gender/lgbtqia-queer-community-on-tiktok-ban. Accessed July 2, 2020.

Rashmi, M. 2019. "Mobile Phones and Changing Media Consumption Practices in Bangalore." PhD Diss., Bangalore: Manipal Academy of Higher Education.

Roy, Shreyashi. 2020. "TikTok Unveils Features to Tackle Its Fake News Problem." *The Quint*. April 30. https://www.thequint.com/news/webqoof/tiktok-to-tackle-fake-news-after-surge-in-misinformation-over-covid-19. Accessed July 2, 2020.

Sanaya, Chandar. n.d. "These Statistics Illustrate the Amazing Popularity of TikTok in India." *Scroll.In*. https://scroll.in/article/942852/these-statistics-illustrate-the-immense-popularity-of-tiktok-in-india. Accessed January 10, 2021.

Schuppli, Susan. 2020. *Material Witness: Media, Forensics, Evidence*. Cambridge, Mass.: MIT Press.

Shalkie. 2020. "Ban on TikTok Is a Huge Blow to Influencers." *Deccan Chronicle*. July 1. https://www.deccanchronicle.com/lifestyle/culture-and-society/010720/ban-on-tiktok-is-a-huge-blow-to-influencers.html. Accessed January 10, 2021.

Shaviro, Steven. 2010. *Post-Cinematic Affect*. Winchester, UK: Zero Books.

Shaviro, Steven. 2013. "Accelerationist Aesthetics: Necessary Inefficiency in Times of Real Subsumption." *E-Flux* 46: 1–9

Shaviro, Steven. 2015. *No Speed Limit: Three Essays on Accelerationism*. Minneapolis: University of Minnesota Press.

Shukla, Pankhuri. n.d. "How TikTok's 'Cringe' Empowered Indians More Than FB or Insta." *Quintype*. https://www.thequint.com/neon/hot-take/tik-tok-ban-empowered-indians-more-than-facebook-instagram. Accessed July 2, 2020.

Siegert, Bernhard. 2015. "Media after Media." In *Media after Kittler*. Ed. Eleni Ikoniadou and Scott Wilson, 79–91. London: Rowman and Littlefield.

Simondon, Gilbert. 2017. *On the Mode of Existence of Technical Objects*. Trans. Cecile Malaspina and John Rogove. Minneapolis: University of Minnesota Press.

Snigdha, Poonam. 2019. "How India Conquered YouTube." *Financial Times*. March 14. https://www.ft.com/content/c0b08a8e-4527-11e9-b168-96a37d002cd3. Accessed January 14, 2021.

Srivastava, Srishti. 2020. "Stars of TikTok, Safe Haven for Artistes, Voices on India's Margins, Speak Out on Sudden Ban." *The Wire*. July 1. https://thewire.in/culture/chinese-apps-ban-tiktok-stars. Accessed January 21, 2021.

Steyerl, Hito. 2009. "In Defense of the Poor Image." *E-Flux Journal* 10, no. 11. https://www.e-flux.com/journal/10/61362/in-defense-of-the-poor-image/.

Stiegler, Bernard. 1998. *Technics and Time*. Stanford, Calif.: Stanford University Press.

Stiegler, Bernard. 2010. *For a New Critique of Political Economy*. Cambridge: Polity.

**54**    Stiegler, Bernard. 2013. "The Pharmacology of Poststructuralism: An Interview with Bernard Stiegler." In *The Edinburgh Companion to Post-Structuralism,* 489–505. Edinburgh: Edinburgh University Press.

Stiegler, Bernard. 2019. *The Age of Disruption.* Cambridge: Polity.

Sundaram, Ravi. 2009. *Pirate Modernity: Delhi's Media Urbanism.* Routledge Studies in Asia's Transformation. New York: Routledge.

Sundaram, Ravi. 2015. "Publicity, Transparency, and the Circulation Engine: The Media Sting in India." *Current Anthropology* 56, no. S12: S297–305.

Tanvir, Kuhu. 2013. "Pirate Histories: Rethinking the Indian Film Archive." *BioScope: South Asian Screen Studies* 4, no. 2: 115–36.

Telecom Regulatory Authority of India. 2020. "Highlights of Telecom Subscription Data as of 31stMay, 2020." https://trai.gov.in/sites/default/files/PR_No.62of2020 .pdf.

Tiwary, Ishita. 2018. "Analog Memories: A Cultural History of Video in India." PhD Diss., Jawaharlal Nehru University.

Warner, Michael. 2002. "Publics and Counterpublics." *Public Culture* 14, no. 1: 49–90.

Weizman, Eyal. 2014. "Introduction: Forensis." In *Forensis: The Architecture of Public Truth,* 9–32. Berlin: Sternberg Press.

Zhang, Xiaoxing, Yu Xiang, and Lei Hao. 2019. "Virtual Gifting on China's Live Streaming Platforms: Hijacking the Online Gift Economy." *Chinese Journal of Communication,* 12, no. 3: 340–55.

Zhang, Zongyi. 2021. "Infrastructuralization of Tik Tok: Transformation, Power Relationships, and Platformization of Video Entertainment in China." *Media, Culture & Society* 43, no. 2: 219–36.

# 3

# Oneirogenic Innovation in Consciousness Hacking

**Aleena Chia**

Lucid dreaming is an altered state of consciousness. It is a phenom-enon where people are conscious they are dreaming while they are dreaming. Lucid dreamers may even have some control over their dream narratives, characters, and environments. These kinds of dreams are experienced in culturally contingent ways depending on whether dreaming is understood primarily as a neurological epiphenomenon, spiritual essence, or resource for personal transformation (Lohmann and Dahl 2014). Whether dreams are understood as waste, essence, or resource, lucidity requires practice. This "dreamwork" of incubating and interpreting dreams takes the form of cognitive, communicative, and pharmacological techniques across different cultural traditions. Dream-potentiating substances—known as oneirogens—are used in dreamwork and may take the form of herbs, nutritional supplements, or drugs (Toro and Thomas 2006). This chapter explores lucid dreaming oneirogens that claim to cut through the work of dreamwork by incorporating ingredients from pharmacological cognitive enhance-ments for nonmedical use known as nootropics.

Dream Leaf is an oneirogen that is taken in two stages: one pill before bed to delay rapid eye movement (REM) sleep and another pill after a few hours to stimulate lucidity and increase dream recall. Combining herbs commonly used for sleep and dream enhancement such as mugwort with psychoactive ingredients for augmenting memory such as Huperzine-A and alpha-GPC, Dream Leaf has been marketed as "a smarter way to lucid dream." Citing Stephen LaBerge, a pioneering psychophysiologist of dreaming, Dream Leaf's website maintains that lucidity in dreaming not only promotes personal growth and creative problem solving, it also contributes to self-mastery (Dream Leaf 2020a). Evoking the mythos of Morpheus's iconic initiation of Neo to psychic awakening in the science fiction film *The Matrix* (1999), Dream Leaf's capsules are colored blue for modulating one's sleep and red for "waking up" in one's dreams.

Lucidity is a framework for commandeering autonomic mental processes to level up in waking and dreaming life. The pharmacological induction of lucidity aligns with "Consciousness Hacking": practices that operationalize an engineering mindset to prime the mind for mystical experiences in a quest to optimize the self (Reagle 2019). Although seemingly esoteric, Consciousness Hacking is a feature of Silicon Valley innovation practices, which rationalize lucidity and other altered states for their noetic experiences of cosmic unity (James 1902). Drawing from online promotion of lucid dreaming nootropics and Consciousness Hacking communities of practice, this chapter shows how the instrumentalization of dreams' noetic qualities within the context of New Age technospiritualities is part of post-Fordist innovation practices.

Oneirogenic innovation—using lucid dreams to seek solutions to waking problems—attempts to routinize creativity neuronally by synthesizing Romantic ideals of originality and emergence with Fordist principles of rationality and reliability. Within the technopharmacology of oneirogenic innovation, neurocentrism— the reduction of complex subjective and cognitive processes to neurobiology—combines with an engineering mindset that puts outcome over process. What arises from this confluence of the spiritual, neural, and technological is a worldview that cuts through the contemplative processes of individual minds and deliberative processes of what is imagined as a social brain. What matters in the Consciousness Hacking worldview are not experiences and explanations but actions and outcomes that can be measured, analyzed, predicted, and optimized. By showing how this worldview underscores specific practices of self-optimization and general principles of behavioral analytics, the case of dream nootropics maps the ideological overlaps between innovation in Silicon Valley and datafication in platform capitalism.

## This is Your Brain on Dreams

> There is no simple surefire way of achieving creativity. Few if any can call upon it at will, and many might find it impossible to invoke. This is, in no small part, because creativity requires a distinct neurophysiological brain state for which there is no simple mental switch. (Stickgold 2019, 145)

Dreams have long been associated with creativity. In *The Committee of Sleep: How Artists, Scientists, and Athletes Use Dreams for Creative Problem-Solving—and How You Can Too,* evolutionary psychologist Deidre Barrett (2001) retells stories of dreams that reportedly helped writers like Mary Shelley and musicians like Paul McCartney create masterpieces. Barrett describes how Dimitri Mendeleev struggled to find a way to classify chemical elements based on their atomic weight and valence. One night after working on the problem, he had a dream of a table where all the elements fell into place, which he recorded immediately after awakening. He reported that this recalled dream image only required one correction before its final form as what we now know as the periodic table of the elements. In *Why We Sleep: The New Science of Sleep and Dreams,* neuroscientist Mathew Walker (2017) explains that the dreaming mind is able to creatively synthesize information and solve problems in a way that eludes the wakeful mind because it makes different mnemonic connections. Whole-brain functional magnetic resonance imaging (fMRI) visualization shows that REM sleep—a phase when dreams often occur—is characterized by relatively pronounced activity in the brain's visual, motor, emotional, and autobiographical memory regions; this is accompanied by less-pronounced activity in regions that control rational thought. Instead of seeking out logical or hierarchical connections between concepts, REM dreaming relates new information to the entire back catalog of existing memories, thereby forging associational links between distant and disparate sets of knowledge. Walker calls dreams' access to diverse combinatorial possibilities "ideasthesia":

> We awake with a revised "Mind Wide Web" that is capable of divining solutions to previously impenetrable problems. In this way, REM-sleep dreaming is informational alchemy. From this dreaming process, which I would describe as ideasthesia, have come some of the most revolutionary leaps forward in human progress. (2017, 219)

Dreaming facilitates the novel combination of existing ideas because it is a biochemical state that is relatively disinhibited from everyday logic, social convention, and sensory stimuli (Barrett 2007). When we dream, the networks of the brain that are associated with executive functioning are dampened, while brain areas associated with emotion are activated (Hurd and Bulkeley 2014). Without the censorship of streamlined neural networks and their tendency toward automated behavior, creative associations flourish in the dream state. In *The Runaway Species: How Human Creativity Remakes the World,* composer Anthony Brandt and neuroscientist David Eagleman (2017) state that humans have an improvisational neural architecture: this supports streamlined neural networks for efficiency, automated behavior, and habits; this also supports arborescent neural networks for flexibility, mediated behavior, and is the neurological basis of creativity. According to Brandt and Eagleman, innovative thinking across artistic, architectural, scientific, and technological fields emerges from practices—and underlying cognitive processes—that combine automated behavior that consolidates expertise with mediated behavior that generates novelty.

Pharmacological oneirogens draw on this popular neuroscientific imaginary to promote the mind as a cognitive wellspring to be plumbed and tapped through the medium of lucid dreams. For example, Dream Leaf's blue and red pill combo claims to "unlock highly creative dreams" (Dream Leaf 2020b) by bypassing the linear thought processes that usually govern our minds during waking life (Hermansen 2016a). Another supplement, LucidEsc offers that lucid dreaming is "not only a liberating and fun experience, it acts as a gateway to finding the answers to our deepest questions" (ViviDream 2020). Nootropics for memory and focus like Alpha BRAIN also promote lucid dreaming as one of its benefits. Like Dream Leaf and LucidEsc, Alpha BRAIN contains the ingredient Huperzine-A, which raises levels of neurotransmitters in the brain for improved memory. Extolling the perks of lucid dreaming, Alpha BRAIN advertises that "in a lucid dream you can fly, kick ass, create art, solve problems" (Onnit, n.d.).

The neurophysiological state for creativity correlates with REM sleep and dreaming, as well as introspective cognitive processes such as mind-wandering or daydreaming, which activate what is known as the brain's default mode network (DMN) (Raichle 2019). During these times, the hyperassociative processes needed to recombine existing memories into novel insights are routinely active. The default mode network denotes a set of brain regions that have high levels of metabolic activity during resting states. Even when not actively focused on specific tasks or current perception, our brains are still generating fleeting mental representations about our memories, our sense of self, and our possible futures. However, like dreaming, the cognitive processes of daydreaming or mind-wandering that activate the DMN are only partly conscious and not reproducible at will (Bruder 2017). Like dreams, DMN states are internally oriented and relatively disassociated from sensory stimulation (Nir and Tononi 2010). Given the significant overlaps between REM and the DMN that show up in neuroimaging studies (Stickgold 2019), some psychologists have theorized that the default network may be a neural substrate for dreaming

(Domhoff 2011). Sleep researcher Robert Stickgold (2019) explains that REM sleep is such a fertile source of creativity because it allows us to explore weak associations that occasionally surface in our dreams. Even without remembering these dreams, creative associations made by the dreaming brain are primed for reactivation and rediscovery when we are awake. However, as Stickgold laments in the opening quote of this section, there is no simple mental switch to turn on creativity in the brain. This is because the thoughts and images from REM dreaming and DMN daydreaming ebb and flow without conscious intent or control, except in the case of lucid dreaming. Experimental psychologists Voss, Holzmann, and Hobson (2009) found out that these areas of the brain that are usually latent during REM were active during lucid dreams, which can be considered as a "hybrid state of consciousness" that combines elements of waking and sleeping cognition.

Lucid dreaming has been verified in lab settings by correlating electroencephalographic (EEG) measurements of REM sleep with physiological (LaBerge 1980) and fMRI indications of lucidity (Dresler et al. 2011). Lucid dreaming is not as rare as one might imagine: according to representative surveys of German adults, about half report having at least one lucid dream (Schredl and Erlacher 2011). Euro-American dream cultures have developed a variety of techniques to incubate lucid dreams, which range from setting an intention before bed to sleep wearables with transcranial direct or alternating current stimulation.[1] Incubation is not uncommon among creative professionals. For example, in their survey of successful filmmakers attending the Sundance Film Festival, Pagel, Kwiatkowski, and Broyles (1999) found that, compared to the general population, directors, screenwriters, and actors reported higher levels of dream recall and use of dreams for waking problems. The incubation of dreams for creativity is easier for the average person to achieve as compared to lucid dreams (Paulson et al. 2017). In their overview of lucid dreaming incubation, sleep researchers Appel, Pipa, and Dresler (2017, 8) conclude that "none of the psychological, pharmacological, or technical

induction techniques developed so far induces lucid dreams
both reliably and safely on demand." Incubating lucidity is a hard
problem to solve, but thankfully, there's a pill for that.

For the price of US$29.99, nootropics like Dream Leaf promise
oneironauts a thirty-night pass to this hybrid state of consciousness where the elusive ideasthesia of REM and DMN states can be
controlled and retained. "Dream Leaf helps you create the right
neural environment for lucid dreaming to take place. It also helps
you recall your dreams better and actually increases your dream
creativity . . . Best of all, you'll start seeing results with Dream Leaf
in less than a week simply by following the directions" (Dream
Leaf 2020b). Dream Leaf works by taking the blue and red pill four
hours apart to prime two different phases of sleep. The blue pill
contains the herbs mugwort for vivid dreaming and valerian root, a
sleep aid that promotes deeper non-REM sleep for the first phase
of the night, which makes it faster to attain REM dreaming cycles
in the second phase of sleep. The red pill uses Huperzine-A and
choline bitartrate to increase levels of acetylcholine, a neurotransmitter that connects dreaming thoughts to waking memories. The
final ingredient, alpha GPC, also allows acetylcholine to accumulate
at higher levels and is known to boost cognitive functions such
as rational thinking. Together, these red pill ingredients improve
chances of lucidity in the second phase of sleep by delaying the
breakdown of acetylcholine, thus counteracting the normal loss
of consciousness during dreaming. These red pill ingredients are
nonprescription acetylcholine esterase inhibitors that are commonly used in nootropics for boosting waking memory and mental
performance.

Within the popular imaginary of pharmacologically enhanced
creative dreaming and oneirogenic innovation more generally,
the goal is never to dream in and of itself. The goal is to use
dreaming for wakeful ideation, but even this is a means to the end
of "awakening": the realization of the perspectival nature of the
human experience that is mediated by a neuronal understanding
of the self. Oneirogenic innovation can be contextualized through

the community of practice known as Consciousness Hacking, which crystallizes this neuronal worldview where the self is flexible, optimizable, and suffused with a promiscuous form of spirituality.

## The Transcendence Industries

> After this, there is no turning back. You take the blue pill—the story ends, you wake up in your bed and believe whatever you want to believe. You take the red pill—you stay in Wonderland and I show you how deep the rabbit-hole goes.

This is a quotation from the film *The Matrix* (1999) of Morpheus offering the protagonist, Neo, a choice to stay ignorant or witness the truth of his existence in a dystopian world where humans are enslaved from cradle to grave in a simulated reality. Morpheus's words are quoted by Dream Leaf to describe lucid dreaming as a fully sensorial simulation that, like the Matrix, you can learn to control (Hermansen 2016b). These claims of radical empowerment—while hyperbolic—crystallize a way of thinking in the innovation industries, where getting ahead is not a matter of shifting gears but shifting paradigms. Like *The Matrix,* the sensorial fidelity of lucid dreams helps us realize that whether asleep or awake, all experience is mentally simulated. This paradigm shift is not just mental or neurophysiological but existential, and is referred to in lucid dreaming communities of practice as "awakening."

Matt, a lucid dreaming content creator with more than 61,000 subscribers, offers that beyond using lucid dreaming for entertainment, therapy, or creativity, its true potential is as a way to understand consciousness to control our urges, drive our behavior, and awaken in our real life (Tipharot 2017). This begins from the realization that lucid dreaming is a fabrication of our minds, which leads to questions about the nature of reality and the role of perception and intention in waking experience. Once we learn to control our dreams, we can learn to control our selves. Taking this a step further, Dream Leaf advocates for "the power of conscious living": once you align your autonomic thoughts and behaviors with conscious intentions, "you will slowly start to see that your behavior is creating the reality you want" (Hermansen 2016c). This focus on intentionality marks lucid dreaming as a contemplative practice along a continuum with meditation. Indeed, experimental psychologist Jayne Gackenbach (1991) proposes that dream lucidity has psychological and physiological parallels with meditation.

Lucid dreaming's brand of existential awakening is part of broader New Age beliefs adopted by a community of practice known as Consciousness Hacking. Consciousness Hacking started in 2013 as a branding network in Silicon Valley to organize events around the mission to "change, upgrade, adjust our internal operating system" (Consciousness Hacking 2016). It currently operates as a fiscally sponsored project of Inquiring Systems Inc., a nonprofit organiza-tion that manages their tax-exempt status (Inquiring Systems, Inc. 2020). According to Jennifer Dumpert (2019, 182), who has given talks on dreamwork at these events, the goal of Consciousness Hacking is to "find ways to use technology (and other evidence-based tools) as a catalyst for psychological and spiritual growth." As these meetups spread from the San Francisco Bay Area to cities around the world, they have been attended by makers, biohackers, researchers, investors, and spiritual practitioners who experiment with electronic, pharmacological, and contemplative techniques to attain altered states of consciousness.

Consciousness Hacking organized the Awakened Futures Summit in May 2020, a two-day online event featuring talks and discussions on psychedelics, meditation, virtual reality, and transcranial stim-ulation for transcendent experiences (Awakened Futures Summit 2020). Consciousness hackers understand altered states of con-sciousness as neurobiological mediums for mystical experiences that are characterized by what scholars of religion call their "noetic qualities": ineffable yet profound revelatory experiences of the truth of reality (James 1902) that are often accompanied by a sense of merging with the universe into oneness and the experience of a changed sense of self (Blackmore 2017). For example, in the panel

"Journey into Technodelics," speakers cited the thirty-item Mystical Experience Questionnaire (MEQ30) (Barrett et al. 2015) as a way to operationalize noetic qualities by rating how psychedelic experiences accorded with feelings of transpersonal unity or nonduality, well-being, and transcendence of time and space.

In addition to the MEQ30, other attempts have been made by Consciousness Hacking and cognate communities of practice to analyze the phenomenology and neurophysiology of mystical experiences in order to replicate them through drugs and dreams. In *How to Change your Mind,* author and journalist Michael Pollan (2018) states that neuroimaging studies of psychedelic drug use suggest that mystical experiences have distinct neural correlates: a reduction of activity in the DMN. As aforementioned, this network overlaps with REM and is associated with introspective and partially conscious cognitive processes such as mind-wandering and dreaming. Pollan offers that since the DMN is implicated in the mental construct we call the ego, the damping down of this network is experienced phenomenologically as the melting away of the familiar boundaries of self and world, subject and object. Self-reporting on the Shulgin Rating Scale (Shulgin and Shulgin 1991) for psychoactive drug use describes this rare state as a blissful and transcendental feeling of connectedness with both the interior and exterior universes that is not easily replicable with the same drug and dosage. This feeling of "oneness" with our inner world, the universe, truth, time, and space identified by the MEQ30 and Shulgin Rating Scale is a peak experience that consciousness hackers attempt to reverse engineer with more efficiency and consistency.

In Consciousness Hacking, the ends of transcendence justify its technopharmacological means. At the Awakened Futures Summit (2020), neurologist Adam Gazzaley proposed that, while the elements of psychedelic experience may start as a molecule, it is the noetic experience that counts. Similarly, Pollan (2018) emphasizes that it is not the pharmacological effect of the drug itself but the kind of mental experience it educes—involving the temporary dissolution of one's ego—that offers therapeutic, spiritual, or creative advantages. Consciousness hackers believe the insight of transpersonal unity can help humans down-regulate their biologically encoded autonomic and unexamined responses of tribalism, addiction, and hedonism in their interactions online and in person. Like psychedelics, lucid dreaming can be considered what former Consciousness Hacking executive director Joshua Fields (2020) calls "self-transcendence technologies," which "give us experiential insight into our interconnection as a species."

From a phenomenological point of view, dreaming ticks many boxes in the MEQ30 and Shulgin Rating Scale: lucid dreaming tends toward sensory clarity, bodily presence, and an expansive emotional thrill (Tedlock 1999); this may also include feelings of self-dissolving into what has been referred to as an "oceanic boundlessness" (Millière 2017; cited in Sanz et al. 2018). Indeed, in their analysis of descriptions of experiences with psychoactive substances, Camila Sanz et al. (2018) found that self-reports of high lucidity dreams had the most similarity to phenomenological descriptions of the psychedelic lysergic acid diethylamide (LSD). Dream researchers Hurd and Bulkeley (2014) maintain that big dreams—with vivid imagery and intense emotions that reverberate through people's self-narratives and life decisions—often involve feelings of awe and ecstasy, emotional catharsis, and nonordinary states of consciousness such as nonduality. For these and other reasons, consciousness hackers like Dumpert (2019) propose that dreaming is the original altered state.

Awakening to mystical experiences is not the ultimate goal of Consciousness Hacking; rather, professional creativity, spiritual transcendence, and personal transformation loop into each other. In a video interview, Robert Waggoner, author of the popular self-help book *Lucid Dreaming: Gateway to the Inner Self* (2009) discusses how his experience of nondual awareness within a lucid dream of blue dots revealed how energy, matter, and consciousness are interconnected in a "oneness" (Conscioius.TV 2012). Based on interviews with fifty people who self-reported varying degrees of nondual consciousness, well-being researcher Jeffery Martin (2015) suggests that these ineffable states are not visions but feelings of a sense of all-encompassing energy that does not generally involve a personalized deity. In *The Finders* (2019), a self-help book endorsed by alternative medicine advocate Deepak Chopra and Consciousness Hacking's top leadership (Fields 2020), Martin offers practical advice on how everyone can experience nondual consciousness to revolutionize their lives. In the context of Consciousness Hacking, noetic experiences in lucid dreaming are often associated with advancement in creative or cognitive professions. For example, educational content platform Mindvalley (2016)—a regular presence at Consciousness Hacking events—instructs that lucid dreaming cultivates conscious awareness in waking life, which can help to control mind wandering, develop empathy, and synthesize multiple diverse streams of information in creative work.

These examples suggest how Consciousness Hacking—whether through pharmacological modulation of REM for lucidity or technological modulation of the DMN for awakening—applies a rational approach of systematization and experimentation that derives from the hacker mindset to altered states of consciousness. For example, the Awakened Futures conference manifesto uses the language of nootropics to promote "stacking" existing contemplative techniques and novel technology: "Stacking this neural fertility with interventions like meditation, neurofeedback, or forms of stimulation could synergize to give non-linear improvements in consciousness." In *Stealing Fire: How Silicon Valley, the Navy SEALs, and Maverick Scientists Are Revolutionizing the Way We Live and Work,* a book endorsed by Consciousness Hacking (Siegel 2017), journalist Steven Kotler and motivational speaker Jamie Wheal (2017) showcase how Silicon Valley executives and engineers use neurobiological and pharmacological techniques and technologies to hack nonordinary states of consciousness for high performance. For example, instead of laboriously practicing meditation, these executives and engineers use neurofeedback to steer themselves to the same state of mind in a fraction of the time. According to

Kotler and Wheal, tuning these altered states of consciousness with relative precision and accessing them nearly on demand is the key to creative problem solving and high-speed decision making that helps individuals move up the leadership chain.

Decoding the underlying neurobiology of altered states in order to modulate them on demand and at scale is the essence of Consciousness Hacking. In *Hacking Life,* communication scholar Joseph Reagle (2019) demonstrates how this hacker ethos of seeking a quick or clever fix in technical systems is being applied to the improvement of all aspects of life. Life hacking takes this fascination with decoding the underlying rules of systems to find shortcuts in personal productivity, nutrition, fitness, dating, and even the quest for meaning in communities of practice such as Consciousness Hacking. Reagle contextualizes that life hacking is self-help for the creative class, which, in the absence of regimentation at work, seeks a regime of its own to minimize distractions and maximize opportunities. This falls in step with technology researcher Melissa Gregg's (2018) contention that productivity apps cater to the flexible work of the creative class by providing temporal and affective structures missing from professional settings. Hacking one's consciousness for creative problem solving is also part of the rise of innovation consulting: corporate services such as workshops that offer Fortune 500 companies and startups replicable methodologies to quickly and dependably generate insights to demonstrate continual change (Wilf 2018).

In the popular science of dreaming, as in Western modernity more generally, creativity and rules are understood to be antithetical and need to be neurologically hybridized through technopharmacology. Just as innovation consulting routinizes, formalizes, and rationalizes creativity through ritual communicative events such as workshops (Wilf 2018), oneirogenic innovation transforms the unruliness of creativity and the ineffability of transcendence into a manageable and reliable resource. The hacking of altered states of consciousness using nootropics is the latest stage in a sustained coevolution of Silicon Valley and New Age cultures (Turner 2016) and, more generally, a historical grounding of instrumental rationality in religious expectation in the West (Noble 1999).

Anthropologists Lucy Suchman and Libby Bishop (2000) state that the deployment of innovation as a construct is always strategic because it places individual actors in a competitive field of action that necessitates a certain order of response. This competitive field is ever more politicized when innovation practices such as Consciousness Hacking are ideologically linked to personhood. For example, Consciousness Hacking's 10 Seeds of Awakened Futures proselytizes that the innovator's consciousness, intentions, and growth manifests in the essence of their innovation and that "personal development is just as important as the creation itself." Anthropologist Lilly Irani (2018) offers that within the innovation paradigm of "design thinking"—a mix of brainstorming, prototyping, cultural observation, and teamwork skills coached by engineering and business schools—the designer's spiritual and personal integration with their outputs is a pivot of value creation. Design thinking sets up a hierarchy in which product and market strategy are linked to personal biographies and seen as too "creative" to outsource, while industrial and mechanical design and manufacturing functions are rendered easy and interchangeable. These criticisms of innovation as individualistic, exclusionary, and conservative have also been leveled against life hacking (Reagle 2019) and hackers more generally (Coleman and Golub 2008). However, the case of oneirogenic innovation in Consciousness Hacking complicates this criticism by implicating society in the self, and the collective good in contemplative practices.

## Manifesting the Social through the Self

At Consciousness Hacking, it's about inside-out change. It's about realising the problems of the world—from tribalism to trauma to war to climate change—are symptoms of how we are relating to ourselves, each other, and our planet. And that by shifting our interior landscape, both

individually and collectively, we transform the world
around us. (Fields 2020)

It is easy to dismiss consciousness hackers as self-serving individuals chasing a high in order to get ahead. Reagle (2019), for example, argues that life hacking breaks the rules of collective systems for personal advantage without thinking about those who have to pick up the slack of one's productivity or the stuff of one's minimalism. Reagle's analysis suggests that the focus of life hacking on the self creates a kind of tunnel vision that blocks out questions about the system's inequities and how to improve it for everyone. However, Consciousness Hacking's stated goal is not just gadgets or even self-transformation but collective state change. As expressed in the quotation by Consciousness Hacking's former executive director Joshua Fields, change from the inside-out means that social change in public policy, economics, and engineering are downstream of human consciousness. This intention for social change extends to applying "holistic design" and "conscious innovation" principles to Consciousness Hacking's supply chain. Along these lines, the Awakened Futures conference (2020) encourages makers, investors, and users to be mindful and minimize the ecological and ethical costs of their technologies' extractive and exploitive use of natural and human resources.

Consciousness Hacking implicates society in self-transformation, in a way that makes it difficult to disentangle its measures for individualization and its intentions of collectivization. The key to understanding the politics of Consciousness Hacking's "inside-out change" lies in understanding the power of intention. Nowhere is this belief in the power of intention clearer than in lucid dreaming's meta-goal of awakening. For example, Dream Leaf states that by becoming conscious to dream scenarios presented by the subconscious mind and then exerting control over dream actions and even environments, lucid dreaming is a unique opportunity to "create an alternate reality" (Hermansen 2016e). This notion of manifesting a second reality in our dreams goes a step beyond simply awakening in real life by directing autonomic thoughts and behaviors. It goes a step further by rooting dreaming and waking experiences in the brain: "After all, our perception of reality is not reality itself but a neurological expression that originates from the senses, just [like] that which is expressed in our dreams. Did your mind just blow? So did mine" (Hermansen 2016d).

Dream Leaf explains that, while sleeping, the brain is able to powerfully simulate smell, touch, vision, hearing, and taste based on imagination and memory (Hermansen 2016e). In a talk at the Science and Nonduality conference that convenes leaders in science and spirituality in San Jose, pioneering lucid dreaming psychophysiologist Stephen LaBerge (Science and Nonduality 2014) states that, whether dreaming or awake, we do not experience the world but our mental models of the world; therefore, lucid dreaming is a means to grasp the illusory nature of all experience. This sentiment echoes what LeBerge has consistently argued. For example, at the lucid dreaming retreat he organized in Hawai'i, LaBerge offers that the realization that reality is created in the mind "tells you that you have much more power than you'd ever believed before—or dreamt—for changing the world, starting with yourself" (Rock 2004, 169).

Within this worldview, such mental potency manifests not just in the dreaming mind's eye and the waking mind's perspective, but also in the brain's neuronal networks. Wellbeing writer Andrea Rock (2004) points to neuroimaging studies demonstrating that dreaming about doing, seeing, or feeling something fires up the same neuronal networks as waking experiences of the same activity. For example, Dresler et al. (2011) used fMRI brain scans to show how a hand movement registered similar neural activity when it was performed awake and while in a lucid dream. The neural basis of manifesting also applies to the therapeutic use of lucid dreaming. In The Joe Rogan Experience Podcast (2013), journalist Steve Volk describes a powerful lucid dream in which he was able to "manifest" his deceased mother. According to Volk (2011), his dream felt so sensorially real—down to the smell of her shampoo and the warmth of her embrace—that it provided the emotional catharsis needed to work through his grief. Dream Leaf encapsulates that "what we control in our dreams is dependent on the level of consciousness we develop, and its [sic] really quite the same in waking life" (Hermansen 2016f).

This belief in oneirogenic manifesting is far from fringe; it resonates with the popular genre of self-help. For example, "How to Manifest Anything" (Zapata 2019), an article in *O: The Oprah Magazine,* rounds up recent self-help books by Angelina Lombardo (2019), Marla McKenna (2019), and others on visualizing professional, romantic, and financial success in one's mind in order to materialize it in one's life. According to these authors, manifesting channels thoughts, actions, beliefs, and emotions toward the materialization of desired feelings and situations through letters to the universe and vision boards. This belief that we "create our own reality" is also shared by New Age spirituality, a syncretic cultural formation of pagan religions, Eastern philosophies, and occult-psychic phenomena (York 1995). New Age spirituality's message of manifesting encourages that "the world we perceive, either positively or negatively, is a projection of our own consciousness and that we can transform our reality for the better by transforming ourselves internally" (Urban 2015, 226).

The individualism of manifesting can be contextualized by the New Age's defining quality, which sociologist Paul Heelas (1996) calls "self-spirituality": the assumption that the sacred cannot be found out there but must be discovered by exploring one's inner psychic space. Anchoring the diversity of New Age orientations is the belief that society represses our authentic selves and that spiritual insight can recover the perfect sacred essence within ourselves. For example, lucid dreaming nootropics are one of many ways to "tap into your personal spirituality" by interpreting dreams, not as figments of your imagination but as "windows into your inner self" (Hermansen 2016g). Summarizing qualitative studies on alternative spiritualities, Steven Sutcliffe (2014) states that New Age practitioners are more likely to be from middle social classes

vying for status and position in risk societies. New Age practices
align seamlessly with worldly objectives such as good health, self-
confidence, prosperity (Bruce 2002), problem-solving, self-healing,
and personal growth (Aupers and Houtman 2010).

In addition to its more obvious resonances with New Age spirituality, oneirogenic manifesting's condition of possibility is the ideology
of "neurocentrism": the idea of the brain as the foundation of
human nature and social life, and the belief in neuroscience's
ability to reveal profound truths about the self and society (Vidal
and Ortega 2017). This assumption that we can understand the
mind—human beliefs, emotions, and behaviors—in the living brain
has been facilitated by the development of brain-imaging technologies such as computerized tomography (CT) scanning in the 1970s
and magnetic resonance imaging (MRI) in the 1980s. According to
sociologist Nikolas Rose and historian Joelle Abi-Rached (2013), this
visual imaginary was central to the project of neuroscience, which
integrated researchers from disciplines as diverse as psychology
and mathematics in a quest to understand the brain as a way to
intervene in it. This intervention came primarily in the form of
psychiatric pharmacology. Today, drugs developed for the purpose
of treating neuropsychiatric disease are increasingly used for enhancement; these interventions take the form of nootropics such
as Dream Leaf and Alpha BRAIN that adjust brain states chemically
to purportedly make healthy brains better (Farah 2012).

Neuro-enhancement—whether for waking cognition or dreaming
creativity—is based on the neuroscientific imaginary of the brain's
plasticity. Evident in popular neuroscience books on dreaming
and creativity by Walker (2017), Brandt and Eagleman (2017), and
others, discourses of neuroplasticity maintain that the brain is flexible, adaptable, and has an almost unlimited potential to form new
patterns of association. Feminist scholar Victoria Pitts-Taylor (2010)
states that plasticity frames the brain as the ultimate biological resource: an untapped potentiality that must be trained to make new
synaptic connections by arousing new states of consciousness and
inciting new modes of thinking. These discourses of enhancement

and plasticity address the subject through the neoliberal ethics of
personal self-care and responsibility that are linked to modifying
the body. Rose and Abi-Rached (2013, 23) lament that "once more,
now in neural form, we are obliged to take responsibility for our
biology, to manage our brains in order to bear the responsibilities
of freedom."

Against this neoliberal backdrop of self-spirituality and neuroplasticity, the ideology of manifesting comes into focus as a plausible
foundation for Consciousness Hacking's aspiration of "inside-out
change." After all, if manifesting something in the sandbox of our
minds is neuronally equivalent to materializing it in our lives, social
change is merely a cumulative effect of individual transformation.
Like the affective recursion of positive psychology that enjoins
people to feel good about good feelings, Consciousness Hacking's
mode of manifestation "presumes the promissory nature of its
own object" (Ahmed 2010, 8). There is an empty space at the core
of Consciousness Hacking that can be manifested with whatever
feels personally right, good, real, and divine. Lucid dreamers
refer to this simply as "the void": minimalistic dreamscapes that
are sensorial and geometric instead of representational (Johnson
2014). Like self-help writer Robert Waggoner's (2012) dream of blue
dots, lucidity's void holds promises of spiritual revelation, neural
flexibilization, and creative inspiration. The promissory plasticity of
the void absolves consciousness hackers from the promiscuity of
manifestation and its conflation of individual transformation with
social change. Understanding Consciousness Hacking's void provides critical insight into the unexamined spaces at the intersection
of neuroculture and platform capitalism, where instead of human
transcendence, human intention is bypassed.

## Bypassing the Mind through the Brain

The neuroculture of lucid dreaming and the data culture of social
media share an operational premise. In the case of dreaming, the
variegated narratives of our subconscious and meanings of our

transcendence are equally legitimate and beyond verification. In the case of platform capitalism, the diverse representational and semantic content of our online activity are equally productive and beneath interpretation. For example, social media platforms don't care about the complex reasons *why* we like someone; platforms do care about our dating patterns that can be predicted by tracking our engagement metrics (Andrejevic 2020). Science and technology studies researcher Johannes Bruder (2019) contextualizes that the neuroscientific reduction of the social subject to its cerebral substrate is informed by the experimental stimulus-response paradigm rooted in the behaviorist influence on twentieth-century psychology. The behaviorist roots of the stimulus-response paradigm proliferates in A/B testing that platforms undertake to optimize engagement. In the cases of neuroculture and platform capitalism, the interpretive and causal qualities of dreaming and communicating are operationally irrelevant; relevance is to be found in pharmacological and design inputs, creative and engagement outputs, and their modulation by physiological and computational correlates. This bypassing of subjectivity in neuro- and data cultures can be traced to the dialectic of media forms and representations, and shifting understandings of what counts as a medium and what is designated as content.

As New Age spirituality made its way through seventies psychedelia and the California bohemia, tensions between neuroscience, psychology, and mysticism became redescribed through tools, techniques, and technologies: this is how religious studies scholar and technology writer Erik Davis (2019) describes what he calls the "consciousness industry." Consciousness Hacking emerged from this confluence of esoteric rituals and pragmatic procedures; what mattered in the experimentation with subjectivity was not how or why but whether a procedure could produce visionary experiences. According to Davis, consciousness itself was imagined as a kind of medium or interface that different kinds of information and sensations could plug into. Citing the popular influence of Marshall McLuhan on the consciousness industry, Davis (2019, 79) encapsulates: "If the medium was the message, then for many seekers and psychonauts, consciousness became the ultimate medium."

What is bypassed in Consciousness Hacking's modeling of the mind as a medium for brain states like REM and the DMN is the representational content of dreams, transcendence, and their politics. For example, Dream Leaf's blog has very few descriptions of dream content; most posts encourage readers to use lucidity to manifest their own desires—whether productive, hedonistic, or contemplative—in their dreams and life. Similarly, the punchline to Volk's dream about his dead mother was not the meaning of the dream itself but the fidelity of its manifestation and effectiveness of its catharsis (The Joe Rogan Experience 2013). Furthermore, descriptions of noetic experiences in Wagonner's dream of blue dots (Conscious.TV 2012), or the MEQ30 (Barrett et al. 2015) do little to convey the interpretive meanings of mystical experiences. This ambiguity is compounded by the nature of noetic experiences, which are individual, isolated, and unexpected. Based on her ethnography with New England mystics, Courtney Bender (2010) offers that the meanings of these experiences are open to recursive interpretation and resistant to sociological falsification.

This tendency toward blackboxing the spiritual experience from collective contemplation is compounded by the New Age's perennialism: the belief that different religious traditions are equally valid, because they all essentially worship the same divine source that emanates throughout the cosmos and the human body (Aupers and Houtman 2014). This perennialism helped New Age spirituality integrate diverse religious, philosophical, and psychological ideas and practices, as well as to cohere as a movement that was individualistic and decentralized (Urban 2015). Nonetheless, what we think of as spiritual is not a neutral phenomenological description but "is actively produced within medical, religious, and arts institutions, among others" (Bender 2010, 23).

This chapter has argued that the use of lucid dreaming nootropics for transcendent experiences is actively produced within neuro-

scientific imaginaries, innovation imperatives, and New Age worl-
dviews. The blackboxing of noetic experiences in Consciousness
Hacking is not as straightforward as rationalizing altered states for
self-optimization. For example, the Awakened Futures guidelines
caution participants against "spiritual bypassing" and "hedonic
shortcuts" that hollow out contemplative processes:

> A technology that encourages short-cutting through hedo-
> nism or repression is not the Consciousness Hacking tool
> of the future. That said, we must not conflate improved
> efficacy with bypassing. (Awakened Futures 2020)

Consciousness hackers believe that automating spiritually
awakened brain states do not have to be at the cost of true enlightenment; they believe that the legitimacy of numinous states
of consciousness does not have to be sacrificed when using them
as mediums for creativity and performance. Commenting on the
paradoxical rise of LSD in the seventies, Davis (2019, 84) states
that the psychedelic drug made varieties of religious or mystical
experiences more visible but, in so doing, contributed to the
"reduction of the soul to the brain." Yet, any logical inconsistencies
or cultural contradictions that arise from this brand of tech naïveté
are smoothed over by the catholic balm of manifestation. This is
the reason why consciousness hackers can share their techniques
of transcendence without debating its purpose; this is also why
Consciousness Hacking can be politically atomistic while sharing
collective practices. In some ways, it is not the technopharmacological automation of altered states but the ideology of manifestation
that is this community's true hack.

Understanding the neurocultural hack of manifestation provides
a critical counterpoint for politicizing the automation of emotions
in virtual reality and the automation of subjectivity in surveillance
capitalism. Media scholar Lisa Nakamura (2020) maintains that
although contemporary VR is presented as an educational tool
for ethical decision making, its true value is as a body hack for the
incitation of morally "good" feelings such as empathy in service

of antiracism and antisexism. "Like meal replacements packs, or other tech industry technologies created to enhance focus by reducing distraction, VR automates the labor of feeling" (Nakamura 2020, 60). Media scholar Mark Andrejevic (2020) makes a similar argument about the promise of automated decision making in data-driven systems, which are premised on preempting human behavior and risk in relation to consumption, mobility, or security. By bypassing human agency, intention, and subjectivity, such decision making "offloads the labor of civic life onto automated systems—it envisions the perfection of social life through its obliteration" (Andrejevic 2020, 109). This obliteration through automation can be traced to early hype about Big Data (boyd and Crawford 2011) epitomized by *Wired* editor Chris Anderson's (2008) proclamation about the "End of Theory": the redundancy of semantic or causal analysis where there is enough data for the numbers to speak for themselves. Informatics scholar Geoffrey Bowker (2014) dispels this hype by emphasizing that data are constituted from interpretive processes such as categorization and links this circumvention of human meaning to the rise of behaviorism in the sciences and neuropharmacology in society.

Nowhere is this bypassing of human subjectivity and foreclosure of human deliberation more salient than in the case of neuromarketing. Legal scholar Mark Bartholomew (2017) offers that the premise of neuromarketing is that observations of brain activity yielded better insights and led to more effective marketing results than any consumer survey. This is done by measuring emotional responses in the brain to stimuli such as commodities and advertisements and segmenting consumers based on the analysis of these somatic markers. Andrejevic (2012) reports that neuromarketing's advocates promote these somatic markers in neurodata as more efficient and effective because it bypasses the slower route of conscious, rational deliberation. Like data-driven decision-making systems, neuromarketing prioritizes correlations of data points for the purposes of prediction, and in so doing blackboxes the problem of causality.

Neuromarketing does away with the model of market research
pioneered by Nielsen, which engaged consumers in some form of
dialogue through written or spoken information. Instead, neuromarketing claims to bypass what people say, to go straight to the source
of what they feel—the brain. According to this rationale, direct forms
of knowledge are contaminated by sociality and, consequently,
language and consciousness (Andrejevic 2012). Bartholomew (2017,
105) contends that by gathering feedback from consumers outside
their awareness, neuromarketing blunts the "democratic promise
of the marketplace [that] lies in the belief that it is responsive to
consumer voice, whether through consumptive choices or more
particularized feedback through traditional market research."

Consciousness Hacking, neuromarketing, and even platform capitalism can be understood as what media scholar Tony Sampson
(2016) calls neurocapitalism: the application of neuroscience findings with technologies to attune working and resting bodies and
minds to the rationalities and regimes of efficiency management.
More generally, neuroculture applies paradigms of neuroscience
across diverse fields such as economics, art, and education. Neuro-
ethicist Martha Farah (2012) states that neuroscience supports a
physicalist view, where human thoughts, feelings, and actions are
the result of physical mechanisms.

In oneirogenic innovation specifically and platform capitalism generally, the automation of emotions, subjectivity, and sociality claim
to provide efficiencies that are hampered by human thought, intention, and deliberation. In a comparable way, the case of Consciousness Hacking automates the neural correlates of transcendence
unfettered by human contemplation. As Bartholomew warns, such
automation comes at the cost of liberal democratic processes and,
ultimately, principles. Neuroculture liquidates our capacity to de-
cide; instead of conscious choices, systems such as neuroeconomics and neuromarketing dissolve human decisions in the calculation
of probabilities (Stiegler 2020) that preempt agency, spontaneity,
and risk in order to map out possible futures (Andrejevic 2020).
Underlying both the design and critique of platform mechanisms

(Van Dijck, de Waal, and Poell 2018) for futures markets of human
behavior (Zuboff 2019) are the familiar reductions of subjectivity
to behavior, minds to brains, experience to mediation. Through
dreaming practices and platform mechanisms, neuroculture is
reframing not just how we understand the human person but also
how we relate to each other in human society.

Farah (2010) states that the field of neuroethics is contemplating
the social and ethical fallout not just of enhancing human brains
but also of the overarching physicalist paradigm in which the
human mind is subject to prediction, influence, and control. Neuroscience is not merely a tool for augmenting humanity but frames
new ways of thinking about humanity, personhood, and their
circumvention (Farah 2012). The datalogical drive to end theory at
best directs policies toward mitigating injustice in computational
decision-making systems, and at worse denies that these injustices
are part of broad social forces (Bowker 2014). In this sense, the
neurocultured platform is a pharmakon: "a remedy that always
contains a poisonous element, and a poison that always holds a
therapeutic virtue" (Stiegler 2020, 173). Although the pharmakon's
toxicity cannot be eliminated, Stiegler maintains in his analysis
of neuroeconomics and neuromarketing that its virulence can be
resisted and that these counterforces constitute the struggle of
knowledge. This chapter calls for culturally informed neuroethics
that questions the physicalist paradigm of neuroscience not just in
its redefinition of the human but also of its reframing of the social.
Philosopher Catherine Malabou (2008) maintains the neuronal is
itself a political and ideological construction and is interdetermined
by economic and social contexts: for example, the plasticity of the
brain naturalizes assumptions and aspirations about flexibility and
optimization in post-Fordist societies. In the case of the consciousness hack, as in the platform mechanism, the biological substrate
of the neuronal self is operationalized in engineering terms
(Bruder 2019): what matters more than the processes of dreaming
and communicating are the measurable outcomes of creativity
and engagement.

**The Neurohumanities of Dreaming**

The case of oneirogenic innovation elucidates how spiritual, technical, and pharmacological modes of contemporary self-making converge in Consciousness Hacking. This chapter analyzed how lucid dreaming nootropics synthesize the worldly goals of creative problem solving with spiritual awakening, thereby modeling the mind through three frames: the design thinking of innovation, the self-spirituality of the New Age, and the neurocentrism of Consciousness Hacking. This chapter argues that while Consciousness Hacking models the mind as a sandbox to master one's thoughts and manifest one's will, capitalist neuroculture models the mind as a black box to be bypassed through the technopharmacological hack. These confluent impulses to manifest and bypass the hermeneutics of dreaming parallel platform capitalism's content-agnostic mechanisms to commodify user engagement. The lucidity of our sleeping dreams and the obscurity of our waking desires are bypassed by a neuroengineering mindset that seeks efficacy over exposition.

Pitts-Taylor (2010, 648) encapsulates that "neuroscience is currently serving undemocratic purposes, but it can be placed at the service of emancipatory politics." Dreams provide an aperture not just to critique the intersection of platform capitalism and neuroculture but also to politicize its dual impulses toward manifesting and bypassing. Dreams have been understood varyingly as waste, essence, and resource. Anthropological approaches have analyzed dreaming as collective portals to spirits and gods in Native American societies (Tedlock 2004). Critical theory has positioned sleep and dreams as interior experiences to be safeguarded from medicalization by brain scanners and optimization by information capitalism (Crary 2013). Like the sleep culture it critiques, critical theory's understanding of dreams as the latent essence of human subjectivity positions dreaming at the margins of Western culture as a dormant, passive, and negative space to be instrumentalized for waking functions (Fuller 2018). Both sleep culture and its critique draw from intellectual and popular ideas about the brain as a wellspring of primal energy to be channeled toward different ends.

However, dreams are not just a neurobiological medium for creativity or productivity; they are an imaginative source of agency. Reporting on the forms and rituals of dreaming on the Greek island of Naxos, anthropologist Charles Stewart (2012) contends that the social resonance of dreams—when various individuals dreamt similar dreams serially and collectively—were a way for people to represent the past and devise exhortations for acting in the present. Stewart (2012, 212) encapsulates that collective forms of action begin in dreams, inciting publics to "work through the problem of agency where a future must be faced using knowledge of the past." Critique of oneirogens must attend to this vitality of dreams; critique of platforms must engage with the imaginative rather than the predictive potentiality of the past; critique of the biological reductionism of neurocentrism must unsettle its own appeals to humanism.

Grappling with humanism in critical interventions to the neuro-centrism of Consciousness Hacking and platform capitalism will require contending with the neurohumanities. The interpretive work of the humanities has traditionally operated from the primacy of human selfhood, human thought, and its relation to the world. This work has also been motivated by human quests for meaning and the aesthetics of worldly coherence. The rise of the neuro-humanities in the work of N. Katherine Hayles (2017) and others has attempted to decenter mentalistic modes of human excep-tionalism by attuning our politics to processes of nonconscious cognition in which human existence falls on a continuum with nonhuman life and material processes. This approach recognizes that all forms of consciousness—human and nonhuman, biolog-ical and technical—emerge from underlying material processes (Hayles 2017). This approach also recognizes that processes of cognition, affect, and aisthesis precede and exceed consciousness (Shaviro 2016).

As the cognitive assemblages of human and nonhuman life as well as material and machine intelligences transform the conditions of our planet, Hayles (2017, 216) emphasizes that "the humanities should and must be centrally involved in analyzing, interpreting, and understanding the implications." The neurohumanistic recognition should not immobilize us from politicizing institutional and popular forms of neuroculture in its pharmacological or computational (Bruder 2019) inflections. Instead of resigning ourselves to these neural forces, we must develop neurological reflexlvlty (Rowson 2011; cited in Rose and Abi-Rached 2013) to attend to neural processes as part of ideological formations as well as cognitive assemblages, not as an engineering problem but as a political imperative.

## Note

1   See Chia (2019) for an analysis of these dream incubation wearables.

## References

Ahmed, Sara. 2010. *The Promise of Happiness.* Durham, N.C.: Duke University Press.

Anderson, Chris. 2008. "The End of Theory: The Data Deluge Makes the Scientific Method Obsolete." *Wired.* June 23. Accessed September 2, 2021. https://www.wired.com/2008/06/pb-theory/.

Andrejevic, Mark. 2012. "Brain Whisperers: Cutting through the Clutter with Neuro-marketing." *Somatechnics* 2, no. 2: 198–215. https://doi:10.3366/soma.2012.0057.

Andrejevic, Mark. 2020. *Automated Media.* New York: Routledge.

Appel, Kristoffer, Gordon Pipa, and Martin Dresler. 2018. "Investigating Conscious-ness in the Sleep Laboratory—an Interdisciplinary Perspective on Lucid Dream-ing." *Interdisciplinary Science Reviews* 43, no. 2: 192–207. https://doi:10.1080/03080188.2017.1380468.

Aupers, Stef, and Dick Houtman. 2010. "Beyond the Spiritual Supermarket: The Social and Public Significance of New Age Spirituality." In *Religions of Modernity: Relocating the Sacred to the Self and the Digital.* Ed. Stef Aupers and Dick Houtman, 135–60. Leiden: Brill.

Awakened Futures Summit. 2020. https://www.awakenedfutures.org. Accessed August 14, 2020.

Barrett, Deirdre. 2001. *The Committee of Sleep: Dreams and Creative Problem-Solving.* New York: Crown.

Barrett, Deirdre. 2007. "An Evolutionary Theory of Dreams and Problem-Solving." In *The New Science of Dreaming, Vol. 3: Cultural and Theoretical Perspectives,* Praeger

Perspectives. Ed. D. Barrett and P. McNamara, 133–53. Santa Barbara: Praeger Publishers/Greenwood Publishing Group.

Barrett, Frederick S., Matthew W. Johnson, and Roland R. Griffiths. 2015. "Validation of the Revised Mystical Experience Questionnaire in Experimental Sessions with Psilocybin." *Journal of Psychopharmacology*. 29, no. 11: 1182–90. https://doi.org/10.1177/0269881115609019.

Bartholomew, Mark. 2017. *Adcreep: The Case against Modern Marketing*. Stanford, Calif.: Stanford University Press.

Bender, Courtney. 2010. *The New Metaphysicals: Spirituality and the American Religious Imagination*. Chicago: University of Chicago Press.

Blackmore, Susan. 2017. *Consciousness: A Very Short Introduction*. Oxford: Oxford University Press.

Bowker, Geoffrey C. 2014. "The Theory/Data Thing Commentary." *International Journal of Communication* 8:1795–99.

boyd, danah, and Kate Crawford. 2011. "Six Provocations for Big Data." In *A Decade in Internet Time: Symposium on the Dynamics of the Internet and Society*. September 21. https://ssrn.com/abstract=1926431.

Brandt, Anthony K., and David Eagleman. 2017. *The Runaway Species: How Human Creativity Remakes the World*. Edinburgh: Canongate Books Ltd.

Bruce, Steve. 2002. *God Is Dead: Secularization in the West*. Oxford: Blackwell.

Bruder, Johannes. 2017. "Infrastructural Intelligence: Contemporary Entanglements between Neuroscience and AI." *Progress in Brain Research* 233:101–28. http://doi:10.1016/bs.pbr.2017.06.004.

Bruder, Johannes. 2019. Cognitive Code: Post-anthropocentric Intelligence and The Infrastructural Brain. Montreal: McGill-Queen's University Press.

Chia, Aleena. 2019. "Virtual Lucidity: A Media Archaeology of Dream Hacking Wearables." *communication+1* 7, no. 2. http://doi: https://doi.org/10.7275/rvqj-n043.

Coleman, E. Gabriella, and Alex Golub. 2008. "Hacker Practice: Moral Genres and the Cultural Articulation of Liberalism." *Anthropological Theory* 8, no. 3: 255–77. http://doi:10.1177/1463499608093814.

Crary, Jonathan. 2013. *24/7: Late Capitalism and the Ends of Sleep*. London: Verso Books.

Consciousness Hacking. 2016. "What Is Consciousness Hacking?" Accessed February 2022. https://www.cohack.org.

Conscious.TV. 2012. "Robert Waggoner 'Lucid Dreaming—Gateway to the Inner.'" Interview by Iain McNay." http://conscious.tv/single.php?vid=1949717468001. Accessed August 14, 2020.

Davis, Erik. 2019. *High Weirdness: Drugs, Esoterica, and Visionary Experience in the Seventies*. Cambridge, Mass.: MIT Press.

Domhoff, G. William. 2011. "The Neural Substrate for Dreaming: Is It a Subsystem of the Default Network?" *Consciousness and Cognition* 20, no. 4: 1163–74.

Dream Leaf. 2020a. "How It works." https://luciddreamleaf.com/pages/how-it-works-2. Accessed August 14, 2020.

Dream Leaf. 2020b. "How Does Dream Leaf Work?" Accessed August 14, 2020. https://luciddreamleaf.com.

Dresler, Martin, Stefan P. Koch, Renate Wehrle, Victor I. Spoormaker, Florian Hols-
boer, Axel Steiger, Philipp G. Sämann, Hellmuth Obrig, and Michael Czisch. 2011.
"Dreamed Movement Elicits Activation in the Sensorimotor Cortex." *Current Biology*
21, no. 21: 1833–37. https://doi:10.1016/j.cub.2011.09.029.

Dumpert, Jennifer. 2019. *Liminal Dreaming: Exploring Consciousness at the Edges of
Sleep.* Berkeley, Calif.: North Atlantic Books.

Farah, Martha J. 2010. *Neuroethics: An Overview.* In *Neuroethics, An Introduction with
Readings.* Ed. Martha Farah, 1-10. Cambridge, Mass.: MIT Press.

Farah, Martha J. 2012. "Neuroethics: The Ethical, Legal, and Societal Impact of Neuroscience." *Annual Review of Psychology* 63, no. 1: 571–91. https://doi:10.1146/
annurev.psych.093008.100438.

Fields, Joshua. 2020. "The State of Consciousness Hacking." *Medium.* https://medium
.com/@joshfields/the-state-of-consciousness-hacking-1ef6667f7cc0. Accessed
August 14, 2020.

Fuller, Matthew. 2018. *How to Sleep: The Art, Biology, and Culture of Unconsciousness.*
London: Bloomsbury Publishing.

Gackenbach, Jayne. 1991. "Frameworks for Understanding Lucid Dreaming: A Review." *Dreaming* 1, no. 2: 109–28. https://doi:10.1037/h0094324.

Gregg, Melissa. 2018. *Counterproductive: Time Management in the Knowledge Economy.*
Durham, N.C.: Duke University Press.

Hayles, N. Katherine. 2017. *Unthought: The Power of the Cognitive Nonconscious.*
Chicago: University of Chicago Press.

Heelas, Paul. 1996. *The New Age Movement: Religion, Culture, and Society in the Age of
Postmodernity.* Oxford: Blackwell Publishers.

Hermansen, Dave. 2016a. "Creativity in Dreams." *Dream Leaf Blog.* December 2.
https://luciddreamleaf.com/blogs/dreaming/creativity-in-dreams. Accessed August
14, 2020.

Hermansen, Dave. 2016b. "Wake Up in Dreams with Lucid Dreaming Supplements."
*Dream Leaf Blog.* December 2. https://luciddreamleaf.com/blogs/dreaming/wake
-up-in-dreams-with-lucid-dreaming-supplements. Accessed August 14, 2020.

Hermansen, Dave. 2016c. "Lucid Living: The Conscious/Subconscious Relationship."
*Dream Leaf Blog.* December 2. https://luciddreamleaf.com/blogs/dreaming/
lucid-living-the-conscious-subconscious-relationship. Accessed August 14, 2020.

Hermansen, Dave. 2016d. "Meditation & Lucid Dreaming." *Dream Leaf Blog.* December
2. https://luciddreamleaf.com/blogs/dreaming/meditation-and-lucid-dreaming.
Accessed August 14, 2020.

Hermansen, Dave. 2016e. "What Is Lucid Dreaming?" *Dream Leaf Blog.* December 2.
https://luciddreamleaf.com/blogs/dreaming/what-is-lucid-dreaming-1. Accessed
August 14, 2020.

Hermansen, Dave. 2016f. "The Thin Little Line between Life and Dreams." *Dream Leaf
Blog.* December 2. https://luciddreamleaf.com/blogs/dreaming/the-thin-little-line
-between-life-and-dreams. Accessed August 14, 2020.

Hermansen, Dave. 2016g. "Elevating Spirituality through Dreams." *Dream Leaf Blog.*
December 16. https://luciddreamleaf.com/blogs/dreaming/elevating-spirituality
-through-dreams. Accessed August 14, 2020.

Hurd, Ryan, and Kelly Bulkeley, eds. 2014. *Lucid Dreaming: New Perspectives on Consciousness in Sleep*. Santa Barbara: Praeger.

Inquiring Systems Inc. 2020. "Fiscal Sponsorship." https://inquiringsystems.org/fiscal-sponsorship. Accessed August 14, 2020.

Irani, Lilly. 2018. "'Design Thinking': Defending Silicon Valley at the Apex of Global Labor Hierarchies." *Catalyst: Feminism, Theory, Technoscience* 4, no. 1: 1–19. http://doi:10.28968/cftt.v4i1.29638.

James, William. 1902. *The Varieties of Religious Experience: A Study in Human Nature*. New York: Longmans, Green and Co. https://doi:10.1037/10004-000.

Joe Rogan Experience, The. 2013. "Joe Rogan Experience #308—Steve Volk." https://thejoeroganexperience.net/episode-308-steve-volk/. Accessed August 14, 2020.

Johnson, Claire R. 2014. "Magic, Meditation, and the Void: Creative Dimensions of Lucid Dreaming." In *Lucid Dreaming: New Perspectives on Consciousness in Sleep*. Ed Ryan Hurd and Kelly Bulkeley, 45-71. Santa Barbara: Praeger.

Kotler, Steven, and Jamie Wheal. 2017. *Stealing Fire: How Silicon Valley, the Navy SEALs, and Maverick Scientists Are Revolutionizing the Way We Live and Work*. New York: HarperCollins.

LaBerge, Stephen. 1980. Lucid Dreaming as a Learnable Skill: A Case Study. *Perceptual and Motor Skills* 51, no. 3 supp12: 1039–42.

Lohmann, Roger Ivar, and Shayne A. P. Dahl. 2014. "Varieties of Lucid Dreaming: An Exploration of Cultural Contingency". In *Lucid Dreaming: New Perspectives on Consciousness in Sleep*. Ed. R. Hurd and K. Bulkeley, 2:23–43. Santa Barbara: Praeger/ABC-CLIO.

Lombardo, Angelina. 2019. *The Spiritual Entrepreneur: Quantum Leap into Your Next Level of Impact and Abundance*. Washington, D.C.: Difference Press.

Malabou, Catherine. 2008. *What Should We Do with Our Brain?* New York: Fordham University Press, 2009.

Martin, Jeffery A. 2015. "Clusters of Individual Experiences Form a Continuum of Persistent Nonsymbolic Experiences in Adults." Center for the Study of Non-Symbolic Consciousness. http://nonsymbolic.org/PNSE-Article.pdf

Martin, Jeffery A. 2019. *The Finders*. Jackson, Wyo.: Integration Press.

McKenna, Marla. 2019. *Manifesting Your Dreams: Inspiring Words of Encouragement, Strength, and Perseverance*. Mukwonago, Wisc.: Nico 11 Publishing & Design.

Millière, Raphaël. 2017. "Looking for the Self: Phenomenology, Neurophysiology, and Philosophical Significance of Drug-Induced Ego Dissolution." *Frontiers in Human Neuroscience* 11 (May): 245. https://doi:10.3389/fnhum.2017.00245.

Mindvalley. 2016. "The Crazy Powers of Lucid Dreaming." YouTube video. September 12. https://www.youtube.com/watch?v=0XUSXz3v3Qg. Accessed August 14, 2020.

Nakamura, Lisa. 2020. "Feeling Good about Feeling Bad: Virtuous Virtual Reality and the Automation of Racial Empathy." *Journal of Visual Culture* 19, no. 1: 47–64. https://doi:10.1177/1470412920906259.

Nir, Yuval, and Giulio Tononi. 2010. "Dreaming and the Brain: From Phenomenology to Neurophysiology." *Trends in Cognitive Sciences* 14, no. 2: 88–100. https://doi:10.1016/j.tics.2009.12.001.

**86**   Noble, David F. 1999. *The Religion of Technology: The Spirit of Invention and the Divinity of Man.* New York: Penguin Books.

Onnit. 2013. "About Lucid Dreaming and How Alpha BRAIN Encourages It." https://www.youtube.com/watch?v=PKI-mb5sLZA. Accessed August 14, 2020.

Onnit. n.d. "Lucid Dreaming Interactive." https://www.onnit.com/lucid-dreaming. Accessed August 14, 2020.

Pagel, J. F., C. Kwiatkowski, and K. E. Broyles. 1999. "Dream Use in Film Making." *Dreaming* 9, no. 4: 247–56. https://doi:10.1023/A:1021384019464.

Paulson, Steve, Deirdre Barrett, Kelly Bulkeley, and Rubin Naiman. 2017. "Dreaming: A Gateway to the Unconscious? Dreaming." *Annals of the New York Academy of Sciences* 1406, no. 1: 28–45. https://doi:10.1111/nyas.13389.

Pitts-Taylor, Victoria. 2010. "The Plastic Brain: Neoliberalism and the Neuronal Self." *Health: An Interdisciplinary Journal for the Social Study of Health, Illness, and Medicine* 14, no. 6: 635–52. https://doi:10.1177/1363459309360796.

Pollan, Michael. 2018. *How to Change Your Mind: What the New Science of Psychedelics Teaches Us about Consciousness, Dying, Addiction, Depression, and Transcendence.* New York: Penguin Books.

Raichle, Marcus E. 2019. "Creativity and the Brain's Default Mode Network." In *Secrets of Creativity: What Neuroscience, the Arts, and Our Minds Reveal.* Ed. Suzanne Nalbantian and Paul M. Matthews, 107–23. Oxford: Oxford University Press. https://doi:10.1093/oso/9780190462321.003.0006.

Reagle Jr., Joseph M. 2019. *Hacking Life: Systematized Living and Its Discontents.* Cambridge, Mass.: MIT Press.

Rock, Andrea. 2004. *The Mind at Night: The New Science of How and Why We Dream.* New York: Basic Books.

Rose, Nikolas, and Joelle M. Abi-Rached. 2013. *Neuro: The New Brain Sciences and the Management of the Mind.* Princeton, N.J.: Princeton University Press.

Rowson, Jonathan. 2011. *Transforming Behaviour Change: Beyond Nudge and Neuromania.* London: RSA.

Sampson, Tony D. 2016. *The Assemblage Brain: Sense Making in Neuroculture.* Minneapolis: University of Minnesota Press.

Sanz, Camila, Federico Zamberlan, Earth Erowid, Fire Erowid, and Enzo Tagliazucchi. 2018. "The Experience Elicited by Hallucinogens Presents the Highest Similarity to Dreaming within a Large Database of Psychoactive Substance Reports." *Frontiers in Neuroscience* 12 (January): 7. https://doi:10.3389/fnins.2018.00007.

Schredl, Michael, and Daniel Erlacher. 2011. "Frequency of Lucid Dreaming in a Representative German Sample." *Perceptual and Motor Skills* 112, no. 1: 104–8. https://doi:10.2466/09.PMS.112.1.104–108.

Science and Nonduality. 2014. "Perception, Dreaming, and Awakening, Stephen LaBerge." YouTube video. February 7. https://www.youtube.com/watch?v=QRs8sR3B2AY. Accessed August 14, 2020.

Shaviro, Steven. 2016. *Discognition.* London: Repeater Books.

Shulgin, Alexander, and Ann Shulgin. 1991. *PIHKAL: A Chemical Love Story.* Berkeley, Calif.: Transform Press.

Siegel, Mikey. 2017. "Stealing Fire." *Consciousness Hacking Blog.* February 20. http://www.cohack.life/posts/stealing-fire/. Accessed August 14, 2020.

Stewart, Charles. 2017. *Dreaming and Historical Consciousness in Island Greece.* Chicago: University of Chicago Press.

Stickgold, Robert. 2019. "Creativity of the Dream and Sleep State." In *Secrets of Creativity: What Neuroscience, the Arts, and Our Minds Reveal.* Ed. Suzanne Nalbantian and Paul M. Matthews, 124–49. Oxford: Oxford University Press. https://doi:10.1093/oso/9780190462321.003.0007.

Stiegler, Bernard. 2020. *Nanjing Lectures (2016–2019).* Ed. Daniel Ross. London: Open Humanities Press.

Suchman, Lucy, and Libby Bishop. 2000. "Problematizing 'Innovation' as a Critical Project." *Technology Analysis & Strategic Management* 12, no. 3: 327–33. https://doi:10.1080/713698477.

Sutcliffe, Steven J. and Ingvild Sælid Gilhus. 2014. "Introduction: 'All Mixed Up'—Thinking about Religion in Relation to New Age Spiritualities." In *New Age Spirituality: Rethinking Religion.* Ed. Steven J. Sutcliffe and Ingvild Sælid Gilhus, 1–16. Milton Park: Routledge.

Tedlock, Barbara. 1999. "Sharing and Interpreting Dreams in Amerindian Nations." In *Dream Cultures: Explorations in the Comparative History of Dreaming.* Ed. David Shulman and Guy G. Stroumsa, 87–103. New York: Oxford University Press.

Tedlock, Barbara. 2004. "The Poetics and Spirituality of Dreaming: A Native American Enactive Theory." *Dreaming* 14, no. 2–3: 183–89. https://doi:10.1037/1053-0797.14.2-3.183.

Tipharot. 2017. "Why Lucid Dream?—7 Reasons to Lucid Dream." February 22. YouTube video, 15.35. https://www.youtube.com/watch?v=224BUhQdBBw. Accessed August 14, 2020.

Toro, Gianluca, and Benjamin Thomas. 2007. *Drugs of the Dreaming: Oneirogens: Salvia Divinorum, and Other Dream-Enhancing Plants.* Rochester, Vt: Park Street Press.

Turner, Fred. 2016. *From Counterculture to Cyberculture: Stewart Brand, the Whole Earth Network, and the Rise of Digital Utopianism.* Chicago: University of Chicago Press.

Urban, Hugh B. 2015. *New Age, Neopagan, and New Religious Movements: Alternative Spirituality in Contemporary America.* Oakland: University of California Press.

Van Dijck, José, Thomas Poell, and Martijn de Waal. 2018. The Platform Society: Public Values in a Connective World. New York: Oxford University Press.

Vidal, Fernando, and Francisco Ortega. 2017. *Being Brains: Making the Cerebral Subject.* New York: Fordham University Press.

Vividream. 2020. "About Us." https://vividream.com/about-us." Accessed August 14, 2020.

Volk, Steve. 2011. *Fringe-ology: How I Tried to Explain Away the Unexplainable—and Couldn't.* New York: HarperCollins.

Voss, Ursula, Romain Holzmann, Inka Tuin, and Allan J. Hobson. 2009. "Lucid Dreaming: A State of Consciousness with Features of Both Waking and Non-Lucid Dreaming." *Sleep* 32, no. 9: 1191–200. https://doi:10.1093/sleep/32.9.1191.

**88**    Waggoner, Robert. 2009. *Lucid Dreaming: Gateway to the Inner Self.* Needham: Moment Point Press.

Walker, Matthew P. 2017. *Why We Sleep: Unlocking the Power of Sleep and Dreams.* New York: Scribner.

Wilf, Eitan Y. 2019. *Creativity on Demand: The Dilemmas of Innovation in an Accelerated Age.* Chicago: University of Chicago Press.

York, Michael. 1995. *The Emerging Network: A Sociology of the New Age and Neo-pagan Movements.* Lanham, Md.: Rowman & Littlefield.

Zuboff, Shoshana. 2019. The Age of Surveillance Capitalism: The Fight for a Human Future at the New Frontier of Power. London: Profile Books.

Zapata, Kimberly. 2019. "How to Manifest Anything: 'The Only Thing Stopping You from Manifesting Your Dreams Is You.'" *O: The Oprah Magazine.* December 17. https://www.oprahmag.com/life/a30244004/how-to-manifest-anything/. Accessed August 14, 2020.

# [ 4 ]

# The Internet of People and Things

### Joshua Neves

> The body is the most basic of all media, and the richest with meaning, but its meanings are not principally those of language or signs, reaching instead into deep wells stocked with vaguer limbic fluids. The body is not one with itself: it is a network.
>
> —John Durham Peters

> *Why is it that we can imagine growing cardiac cells in a lab, but not growing empathy for other human beings in our everyday lives?* For many people, the idea that we can defy politics as usual and channel human ingenuity toward more cooperative and inclusive forms of social organization is utterly farfetched. Thus I am convinced that we must query this faith in biological regeneration that stands alongside an underdeveloped investment in social transformation. *If our bodies can regenerate, why do we perceive our body politic as so utterly fixed?*
>
> —Ruha Benjamin

This chapter explores the mainstreaming of smart technologies and cognitive enhancement. In my larger research, I refer to this mode of networked vitality as *smart bodies.* Smart bodies combine a range of biological and computational purposes—from smart drugs to smartphones—that operate on the logic of optimization and whereby biotechnical reproduction and capital accumulation are spliced in new ways. Drawing on a range of debates about augmentation, resilience, and surplus, my aim is to trace contemporary *neuropolitics*—namely, a set of techniques geared toward hyperbolic performance that generates new thresholds for physical and cognitive (dis)ability and animates uneven geopolitical relations.

I find focusing on the nexus of drugs and devices a useful way to maintain the centrality of the human body as a nodal point within a thicker ecology of development. From stories about parents obtaining off-market Adderall to keep their children competitive, to the current fascination with microdosing as a necessary supplement for dynamic performance in the creative economy, to more mundane forms of nutrition, stimulation, or habituation, we are witnessing an intensification of voluntary and purposeful modes of self-optimization (alongside a concomitant disinvestment in social transformation). My basic assumption is that these biotechnologies must be understood alongside related shifts in the technologies of everyday life: including devices like phones, tablets, TVs, and Fitbits, as well as the broader proliferation of networked sensors. Put differently, while much research on smart technology and algorithmic culture emphasizes machine learning or the Internet of Things (IoT), this chapter examines *the internet of people and things*—refusing the narrow technophilic myth that sees smart tools as working for, rather than *in* or *through* the human body (Neves 2020). This is not simply to say, following John Durham Peters above, that "the body is a network" but also that much can be learned by understanding the network as a body.

## Understanding Technopharmacology

I begin by considering the "neo-McLuhanesque injunction" informing contemporary media theory (Mitchell and Hansen 2010, xxii). What interests me about the reappraisal of McLuhan—for example, in the works Friedrich Kittler and iterations of so-called German media theory (Kittler 1999; Beyes, Conrad, and Martin 2019); W. J. T. Mitchell and Mark B. N. Hansen's critical mediation (2010); Sarah Kember and Joanna Zylinska's "lifeness" (2012, 3); John Durham Peters and varied approaches to elemental media (2016);[1] and even the "radiant infrastructures" examined by scholars like Rahul Mukherjee (2020); or engagements with McLuhan in China and Japan (Han 2011; Steinberg 2017)—is the consolidation of a media paradigm rooted to what McLuhan dubbed "the extensions of

man." Recall the opening gambit in "The Medium Is the Message."
McLuhan writes: "the personal and social consequences of any
medium—that is, of any extension of ourselves—result from the
new scale that is introduced into our affairs by each extension of
ourselves, or by any new technology" (1964, 1). In other words,
what we might lightly term the *externalization thesis*—where media
are "out there," thingly, prosthetic, infrastructural, environmental,
logistical—implicitly and explicitly shapes our metaphors, politics,
and research programs in consequential ways.[2] There are good
reasons for this and of course a good deal more complexity than
I am able to treat here. My simple claim is this: the externalist
tendency covers over other and lesser attended vectors—including
those that are important for apprehending technopharmacology as
an embodied phenomena.

Let me briefly sketch some aspects of this tendency before sug-
gesting an alternative tack. First, neo-McLuhanesque scholarship
has moved beyond tired debates between technological deter-
minism, on the one hand, and theories of media use or practice,
on the other, as what matters when we try to understand media.
Indeed, multiple veins of contemporary media theory have sought
to reinterpret McLuhanist insights at a more basic or banal level.
"'Understanding media,'" as Mitchell and Hansen put it in their
Introduction to *Critical Terms for Media Studies,* "does not mean
just (or primarily) understanding individual mediums—electricity,
the automobile, the typewriter, clothing—but rather something
like *understanding from the perspective of media*" (xi). Paraphrasing
Friedrich Kittler's well-known aphorism, they conclude: "rather
than *determining* our situation . . . media *are* our situation" (xxii). In
this way the authors reject any simplistic sense of our "prosthetic
being" (e.g., as discrete or singularly determined) and emphasize
the importance of relationality—that is, mediation itself—to the
emergence of human life (xii). This imbrication of the human and
the technical sees the body as neither a preexisting technology nor
as a simple receiver of signals. Instead, the body "comprises the
non–self-sufficient 'ground' for all acts of mediation, including those

(the vast majority of mediations) that expand its agency beyond the 'skin'" (xiii). Here I simply want to observe the forked path suggested by this characterization. The body is at once essentially relational and yet, in the same breath, this relationality is given a clear vector. It extends, projects, radiates.

Tied to McLuhan by both a publication date, 1964, and its reverberating impact, is a parallel approach suggested by the French paleontologist André Leroi-Gourhan's *Gesture and Speech.* The latter also serves as a catalyst for Bernard's Stiegler's focus on the "co-originarity" of humans and techne in *Technics and Time* (Leroi-Gourhan 1964; Stiegler 1998). If *Understanding Media* consolidated the sense of media technologies as extended or prosthetic organs, Leroi-Gourhan's *Gesture and Speech* tracks the inverse: the ways that bodily organs can be understood as expanded technologies (Peters 2016, 16). Peters summarizes Leroi-Gourhan's contribution as follows:

> Leroi-Gourhan showed the coevolution of the human musculoskeletal form with techniques such as walking, gathering, chewing, speaking, drawing, writing, and remembering. He understood that the intertwinement of embodied practice and technical objects went from cranium to toe. For him the human condition was defined precisely by our standing on two feet—and by our consequent impossibility of separating nature and culture. (17)

As above, Leroi-Gourhan, via Stiegler, Peters, and others, provides a complex model of coevolution or feedback—where, for example, walking and chewing shape and are shaped by the very bones of the body. What interests me about this framing, as with McLuhan above, is how it both indicates a wide range of conceptual possibilities and yet seems to have sedimented in ways that limit the contemporary media imagination. From tools to environments to platforms, much of our thinking about media is quick to seek out that which is outside, below, or beyond. The refrain: media extend, ground, surround, organize. Without overstating my case, and recognizing the importance of extensions—from hard drives and smartphones to undersea cables and neural networks—I want to suggest a simple inversion of McLuhan's essentially centrifugal spark. It is time we give more critical attention to *the intensions of (hu)man.*[3] Put differently, instead of amputation (McLuhan's antonym) or nature (a common inversion of prosthetic or artificial), intension suggests centripetal qualities or processes of *coming into the body.* In what follows, I examine media technologies as part of a larger history of stimulants and other pharmacological processes, including smart drugs, transcranial direct current stimulation (tDCS), blood transfusions, digital medicine, among other supplements or techniques. This is not only to shift attention from exteriorization to processes of *ingestion, absorption, inhalation, injection,* and so on, but also to revisit the pharmakon (Derrida 2000; Rinella 2010; Stiegler 2010)—the capacity of drugs and other technologies to be beneficial and harmful at the same time—from the vantage of our present dilemmas.

## The Polypharmacy

If, as Wolfgang Schivelbusch observes, the cigarette was the symbol of modernity and "embodied speed, transience, the hectic big city, and advertising," then smart drugs may be the figure of the current phase of cognitive capitalism (Shivelbusch 1992, 185). Indeed, Schivelbusch both draws our attention to a longer history of neurocentrism, where the brain overshadows the body, and traces how everyday stimulants like coffee, tea, and tobacco have long been used to create dispositions for mental work, among other moods or microvitalities (see also Chia in this volume). On the polypharmacy of caffeine and nicotine, he writes:

> Although since the seventeenth century tobacco and coffee had been considered particularly suitable for the intellectually active, their effects stand in remarkable contrast to one another. Tobacco *calms,* coffee *stimulates.* Normally one would assume that these contradictory

qualities cancel each other. The common goal both were used to achieve was the reorientation of the human organism to the primacy of mental labor. The brain is the part of the human body of greatest concern to bourgeois civilization. It alone was developed, cultivated, and cared for in the seventeenth and eighteenth centuries. The rest of the body, necessary evil that it was, merely served as support for the head (110).

Schivelbusch's description of mental labor, harmonized drugs (e.g. coffee and cigarettes), and the superimposition of pleasure and obligation—what he terms "performance-in-the-process-of-enjoyment" (xiv)—are just one thread in a longer history of smart substances. I linger here both to situate the examples that follow and because Schivelbusch's understanding of the ways pleasurable stimulants, intoxicants, and other technologies tie us to society bends the idea of the pharmakon in useful ways. Beyond the classical sense of poison and cure—and the Platonic notion that "the *pharmakon* goes against natural life" (Derrida 1981, 99; original emphasis)—attending technology *and* pharmacology brings into relief emergent tensions between disease and health, smartness and resilience, people and things. This is not simply to say, again drawing on Jacques Derrida's reading of Plato, that "there is no such thing as a harmless remedy" (99) or that the essential ambiguity of drugs is aporetic, an impasse. Instead, my aim here is to draw out the "*productive* potential" of drugs and devices—their capacity to remake bodies, work, and politics in unexpected ways (Persson 2004, 46; Race 2009).

Here I also want to observe that technopharmacology is entangled with a "global shift toward excitants," where stimulants have steadily displaced narcotics (e.g., opioids) as the drugs of choice around the world.[4] In their history of *Narcotic Culture* in China, Dikötter, Laamann, and Zhou trace how opium gave way to tobacco in the early twentieth century, and how later, even with the surge of heroin use in the reform era,[5] amphetamine-type stimulants (ATS), including methamphetamines, have taken center stage as

"consumers the world over [sought] designer drugs more attuned
to new patterns of work and leisure" (2004, 210–11). The latter have
long and complex histories but were used widely by soldiers and
workers during World War II and, following the war, were dumped
on domestic markets to be reimagined as "mother's little helpers"
or as necessary supplements for salarymen in Japan, among others
(Wolkoff 1997; Sato 2008; Andreas 2020). The history of ATS can be
traced back to the Chinese herb *ma huang* (ephedra), a drug used
for thousands of years before being synthesized in 1887 and adopted in medical practice in the 1930s as amphetamine. Alongside
distinct local histories of cannabis, coca, tobacco, and many other
stimulants,[6] the rise of legal drugs like Adderall or illegal drugs like
methamphetamine shore up an *economy of speed.* This "new narco-
capitalism," as Jason Pine describes it, "can give you more energy,
more working hours, *'more life'*" (2007, 360; 2019).

The global surge in stimulant production, distribution, and use is
also tied to the rise of smart and networked devices. This includes
the grey internet, distinct legal geographies, and shifting ideas
about the body and health, as well as intimate connections to
smartphones, algorithmic identities, and cultures of optimization.
This polypharmacy of technology and tonics includes both new and
old habits and objects, as well as the ways they are mixed, sched-
uled, and mutually intensifying. For example, when a session at
the 2018 World Economic Forum held in Tianjin, China, asks "What
If: Smart Drugs Become as Common as Coffee?" it is also asking
about the role of stimulants, and of smartness paradigms more
generally, as practices of everyday life. The panel—which focused
on familiar tensions between therapy and enhancement, individual
rights versus social equity, and smart decisions as opposed to
addictive habits—is emblematic of an increasingly technopharmacological condition. A condition marked not only by the proliferation of digital infrastructures but also the explosion of coffee
consumption in places like China, India, and Indonesia (Harbeck
2019), Attention Deficit/Hyperactivity Disorder (ADHD) diagnoses
and prescriptions worldwide (Smith 2017), nootropics and other

drugs for concentration and productivity (Partridge 2012; Battleday and Brem 2015; Dance 2016), legal and illegal amphetamine (and so-called speed) use around the world (Pine 2019; Andreas 2020), e-cigarettes and vaping (including cannabis), and much else besides.[7] The latter in particular provides an evocative image of the polypharmacy. Leading electronic cigarette brands, like JUUL and RELX, operate as tech start-ups and are now part of the internet of things. Their vaporizers are designed to look like computer flash drives, are charged through USB ports or smartphones, and can be controlled by apps.[8] This allows them to disappear as habitual objects (e.g., as thumb drives, pens, etc.) and to become *smart/drugs* in at least two senses: they are, at once, breathed into the body to foster a desired disposition and, at the same time, communicate with network algorithms and infrastructures.

Consider the at once buoyant and terrifying claim from the CEO of HVMN that "Humans are the next platform" (Morris 2016). HVMN is a Silicon Valley company selling ketone enhancers and nootropic supplement "stacks" that promise to boost energy, focus, memory, metabolism, sleep, and overall brain function.[9] The term *nootropic* (from the Greek: "mind" + "bending") was coined by the Romanian chemist Corneliu Giurgea as a label for Piracetam, a drug he synthesized in 1964, and later associated with increased cognitive ability. Nootropics include a range of naturally occurring and fabricated compounds—including racetams, central nervous system stimulants (like amphetamines, methylphenidate, or even caffeine and nicotine) as well as a wide range of traditional herbs and supplements sold in health food stores around the world—that, while largely unregulated, have become both big business and are important to the life-hacking ethos of the "professional managerial class" (Ehrenreich and Ehrenreich 2013).

In a profile in *New York* magazine titled "The Pill Freaks of Silicon Valley," the company's cofounder, Geoffrey Woo, frames the decision to focus on human optimization crassly. He asks, "where's the next billion dollars of value [going to be] created?" Woo continues:

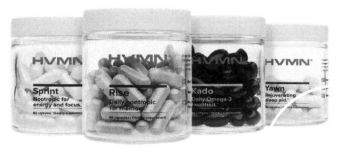

[Figure 4.1]. HVMN's nootropic supplement stacks—sprint, rise, kado, yawn—claim to augment performance by supporting microstates, like focus or rest, as well as overall physical and cognitive health.

What I saw was that the sensors on pure tech are stagnating. Like, people have been complaining about this for the last two or three years—the hardware, the number of sensors on your phone have plateaued. But sensors on the human body were growing really quickly. We're tracking heart rate, we're tracking footsteps, your microbiome is being surfaced up . . . all these things. Pulling data from the human body was now in this explosion phase. (Morris 2016)

Crucial to this explosion is the value of bioanalytics for performance optimization and speculative markets. But beyond the familiar focus on how our clicks and likes are tied to targeted advertising, predictive modeling, and similar nudges or profiles, sensors on the body also tell a different story about the value of our data, energies, and futures. Body sensors fuel an emergent field of computational medicine that, no longer content to merely track and trace, now also intervenes chemically on motor, cognitive, and affective systems (Chatterjee 2004; Zhang 2015). This shift from harm reduction or remedy to perpetual experimentation and self-improvement not only recasts the classical pharmakon by making it chronic, what Joseph Dumit calls *drugs for life* (2010), but also crystalizes a new relationship between Big Data and big pharma.

HVMN is just one example out of countless self-optimization start-ups around the world—from projects centered on nutrition, transfusions, and pills to meditation apps, self-tracking communities, and DIY brain stimulators. It draws our attention less to effective forms of cognitive or corporeal enhancement—the research on smart drugs and trendy diets remains spotty—and more to a new set of expectations and aspirations enunciated by networked life, including its claims on neurological, physical, and affective states. Put differently, HVMN's claim to "relentlessly pursue human optimization" is tied to changing norms about bodily capacity, temporal experience, and the relationship between people and objects. In addition to familiar drugs—like tea to wake, cigarettes to break, alcohol to sleep—so-called smart drugs increasingly partition the daily rhythms of work and leisure into microstates or doses of energy, calm, attention, creativity, and so on. And they do so in concert with an emergent ecology of smart things. This is both to reiterate Ravi Sundaram's claim, in chapter 2, that smartphone videos operate as a cultural narcotic that "fuels the rhythms of everyday life and produces temporal markers of day and night," and to argue that smartness is, at its core, a technopharmacological problem or mandate.

## Brain Games

An open letter in the July 2016 journal of the *American Neurological Association* signals some of the contours of this phenomena. The letter directly addresses "do-it-yourself users of Transcranial Direct Current Stimulation" (tDCS)—a noninvasive procedure that sends electrical current into the brain with the aim of increasing neuroplasticity and thus accelerating the capacity to learn (Wurzman, Hamilton, Pascual-Leone, Fox 2016). While associated with improved cognitive function in some studies, and used as a specialized treatment for brain disease, injury, and psychiatric disorders, what prompted the letter from prominent neurologists is the widespread use of tDCS by amateurs, hobbyists, and otherwise healthy people. This includes hundreds of online videos and forums showing users how to build simple devices and administer current, DIY and hi-tech electrical kits or headsets for purchase on platforms like Amazon and Alibaba, as well as a growing market for related products that promise to boost performance.

One recent and impactful example is Halo Sport's patented brain stimulator. Boasting partnerships with elite sports franchises and Olympic teams (before being discontinued in 2021),[10] Halo Sport promised to "upgrade your brain" and help "just about anyone" learn movement, strength, endurance, and skill faster. Users wear the headset for twenty minutes to "prime" their brain before work-outs, practice, or study. One of many such products, the headset sends a small electrical signal to the motor cortex "putting it in state of hyperplasticity" and readying the brain for "hyperlearning." According Halo's data, regular priming, training, and tracking leads to "45% faster results" and "13% better performance." A common metaphor used in this and similar literature is that of the sprinter. Even a small improvement of a fraction of a second may be the difference between winning and losing. As one user, a pianist, notes in the comments: "Before Halo, I would have said there are no shortcuts to focused practicing. Halo allows you to tune into the body as well as focus on the music at the same time. I'd say my practice has become up to 4X more effective. With Halo, I am able to learn faster and more completely, making the most out of each practice session. I am a fan!" Halo Sport 2.0 sells for $399 online and, in a section of the product's website titled "real science, real results," links to dozens of peer-reviewed studies supporting its safety and effectiveness. While certainly costly and a niche product, it is emblematic of hundreds of similar products and homemade devices in an increasingly crowded neurotech market.

In contrast to the niche market and high cost of Halo Sport, consider a popular amateur video channel (circa 2012) that both documents one user's self-experimentation and teaches others how to make their own tDCS kits. Widely circulated across TV news and documentary media, videos like "Still Zapping My Brain" capture the amateur and experimental nature of the subculture as

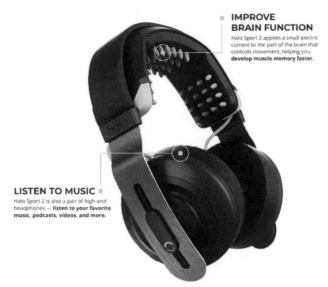

**IMPROVE BRAIN FUNCTION**
Halo Sport 2 applies a small electric current to the part of the brain that controls movement, helping you **develop muscle memory faster.**

**LISTEN TO MUSIC**
Halo Sport 2 is also a pair of high-end headphones — **listen to your favorite music, podcasts, videos, and more.**

[Figure 4.2]. Halo Sport's patented neuropriming system promised to "upgrade your brain." Headsets, which double as headphones, sold online for $399.

well as the many risks associated with DIY brain stimulators. The video, just one example out of thousands of such tube channels, subreddits, self-quant forums, and wellness influencers,[11] gained traction in large part because of how it portrays the haphazard application of electrical current to the brain by healthy and often youthful users. The user in the video, anthonynlee, walks us through the trial and error of his "brain games." It opens: "Hi there, it's me again. So, I have the machine perfected, well almost perfected . . . I mean it's a lot better than it was last time." He continues by noting his struggles to place the sponge electrodes correctly, anxiety over flashes of light, and uncertainty about whether he feels anything. "I imagine over time," the video concludes, "I will start seeing results as far as working memory is concerned . . . I just have to keep playing these games."[12]

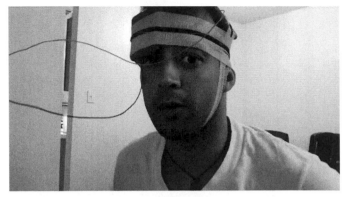

[Figure 4.3]. "Still Zapping My Brain. DIY tDCS Volume Two" (2012) is one of thousands of videos showcasing amateur tDCS experiments.

The image of young people sending electricity from a nine-volt battery into their brain and posting it on social media in the hopes of getting smarter, faster, or more skilled is a telling example of the networked vitalities at issue here. It points to both new desires and demands for heightened capacities, as well as new forms of risk and exposure. These risks are distinct, the scientists state in their open letter, because the risk–benefit analysis for healthy people is different than for those dealing with extreme or life-threatening conditions. Healthy subjects, they assert, "have less to gain, and more to lose." This is one of the chief contradictions associated with the mainstreaming of performance enhancement: it normalizes vulnerability and inequality in the name of human enrichment. At the same time, it exacerbates existing gaps between so-called normal populations and those marked by bodily, cogni-tive, and sensory differences. This has led many pop-tech commen-tators to note that the future will be increasingly defined by gaps between enhanced and unenhanced people—a refrain repeated by texts ranging from the 2011 film *Limitless;* ESPN's six-part documen-tary series *Enhanced* (2018); VICE videos exploring "humanity+" or "Modafinil in India"; the transhumanist documentary *The Future of*

*Work and Death* (2016); and a 2018 documentary about Adderall, *Take Your Pills*; among countless others.

Adderall and transcranial direct current stimulation are just two among many interventions now commonly referred to as "cosmetic neurology"—neurologist Anjan Chatterjee's term for the possibilities and perils of improving cognitive systems, not in disease, but in health (2004). The phrase captures the tensions between the pleasures and demands for self-improvement as well as the gendered dismissal of such practices as merely "cosmetic," narcissistic, or frivolous. Focusing on neuropharmacological interventions, Chatterjee, director of the Penn Center for Neuro-aesthetics, delineates three prospective categories associated with better brains and bodies: "movement, mentation, and mood" (973). Cosmetic neurology thus draws our attention to the mainstreaming of performance-enhancement aids—no longer limited to therapy, professional athletes, or fringe body hackers. These practices work broadly on the body and on embodied networks: cognitive augmentation mingles with improvements in the motor system, mood and affect, as well as a range of technological systems. Put differently, the self-optimization projects of healthy subjects drives both new standards for attention, creativity, vitality, and risk, as well as deep changes in the political economy of the body and qualities of life. As Chatterjee asks, "if we can make better bodies and brains, who gets them?" (971).

As if addressing such divides, Wendy Brown observes that every society consumes the drugs that reflect, in some ways, its political economy and political values. From the nineteenth-century opium of the masses to contemporary antidepressants, antianxiety drugs, and now capacity-enhancing drugs like Adderall, Ritalin, and Modafinil, among other nootropic supplements, illegal stimulants, pills for erectile dysfunction, and the like. The rise of so-called mass cultural doping underscores the everyday substances and supports used by large populations as technologies of advantage, endurance, and survival (Brown 2016). Brown's comment about mass cultural doping echoes Johnathan Crary's worry that what begins as a "lifestyle

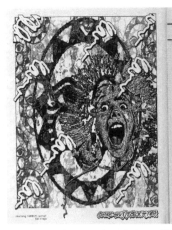

Better Brain Change Through Electricity

# MIND MACHINES TODAY

### by Jay Cornell

*Mind machines — technological devices that affect the mind — have arrived. Although the field is very much in its infancy, it's easy to perceive the outline of a future where these machines will play an important role — extending and expanding our faculties and allowing greater control over our mental states and moods. Recently, Michael Hutchison, author of the definitive book on mind-machine technology -* Megabrain *- hosted a workshop in Silicon Valley. Attendees were treated to hands-on (or is it heads-on?) demonstrations of a dozen gizmos. Jay Cornell is an Oakland-based technophile and assistant publisher of* Gnosis *magazine. Wearing his Reality Hackers beanie, he attended the day-long seminar and issued the following report.*

Remember the hoopla about biofeedback devices in the late '60s? They really could reduce stress and aid meditation, worthy - though not terribly exciting - goals. Then in *Megabrain* I discovered how mutant descendants of biofeedback instruments had been designed to exploit the latest brain research findings and were, among other feats, allevi-

ating pain, curing diseases, sending people on mental trips to other planets, unleashing creativity, raising IQs, and growing hair on the bald. I realized we were in the early stages of yet another Brain Change Revolution.

### MACHINES FOR CHANGING MINDS

This Revolution is in its wild and woolly early stages at the moment. The FDA watches carefully while a few doctors tentatively use some machines for treating stress, relieving pain and aiding wound healing, but these Authorities still pooh-pooh the more extravagant claims and warn against charlatanism. Meanwhile, eccentric experimenters and entrepreneurs are in their basements and garages building machines, just as the mid-'70s hackers built the first personal computers. On the research front, scientists are performing and replicating experiments that overturn long-held beliefs about the brain, and the results are adapted to the next generation of machines. The whole mind machine field is poised to take off. Right now, it's a growing but volatile mixture of scientific research, budding entrepreneurs, in-

REALITY HACKERS 15

[Figure 4.4]. A feature in the 1988 issue of *Reality Hackers* glimpses a longer history of brain-stimulation devices. The magazine, renamed *Mondo 2000* in 1989, was a precursor to *Wired.*

option" will soon become, for many, a requirement (2013, 3). The continued rise of everyday and experimental smart drugs suggest a shift from the therapeutic focus on managing pain, anxiety, or depression toward increased demands for heightened performance or, following transhumanist thinkers, *humanity+.* Contemporary technologies of enhancement represent a complex form of human extraction marked by pharmacological acceleration. Subjects must not only endure intensifying risk and self-responsibility but become newly optimizable and resilient.

My interest here is to consider how "smart drugs," among similar phenomena, are imbricated with the proliferation of other smart technologies—like smartphones, smart homes, smart cities—what Halpern, Mitchell, and Geoghegan call the *smartness mandate,* after IBM's "smarter planet" initiative, to describe "the interweaving of dynamic, emergent computational networks with the goal of producing a more resilient human species" (2017, 107). Put differently, cosmetic neurology and related forms of augmentation are captured and amplified by computer systems in ways that transform both bodies and networks. In what follows, I want to build on Halpern's claim that the goal of smartness is *resilience.* Resilience shores up a set of processes or infrastructures that "can absorb constant shocks while maintaining functionality and organization" (121). It is a mode of embodiment and worldmaking that refuses stability or equilibrium—what we have traditionally understood as key to healthy bodies and ecosystems—and instead embraces permanent optimization and plasticity. This is to say, first, that smartness and the speculative economy manage uncertainty through constant enhancement or update (Chun 2016); and, second, that networked optimization, as mundane pleasures and relentless crisis management, consolidates a distinct and increasingly perilous idea of resilience.

## After Optimization

While the above sections focus on smartness through the lens of drugs and other stimulants or stimulations, smartness is much more often associated with the Internet of Things (IoT), including shifts in cloud and edge computing, machine learning, and 5G infrastructures that are imagined to bring to a new thingly-ness to life. The interweaving of these two senses of "smart"—that is, smart drugs and smart devices—is at the very heart of this chapter's engagement with technopharmacology. Before returning to the question of resilience, I want to pause for a moment to consider the origins, or at least one origin story, of the IoT.

The tech entrepreneur Kevin Ashton is credited with coining the phrase the "Internet of Things" in a 1999 presentation at Proctor and Gamble. He subsequently cofounded the Auto-ID Center at the Massachusetts Institute of Technology, which established global standards for Radio Frequency Identification (RFID), among other sensor technologies. Interestingly, the concept emerged from Ashton's work in the mid 1990s as a brand manager involved in launching the Oil of Olay cosmetic line. Ashton claims to have come up with the idea after visiting a local pharmacy where he noticed that many of his most popular products were out of stock. Further investigation showed that 40 percent of the cosmetics were off the shelves at any given time. He asks: "But why? We had made enough products, but they were sitting in our warehouses, never making it to the empty shelves. And that was a clue: the stores did not know they were out of stock" (Ashton 2015, n.p.) Ashton would go on to associate this problem with inadequate information systems and barcode scanning, but especially with human error. As he notes in recent interviews, this simple observation led to a paradigm shift away from human-entered data—which is "error prone, inexact, and expensive" (Ashton)—and toward sensors that communicated over the internet. He sums up this shift as follows: "The real world contains countless trillions of terabytes of information, and twentieth century computing could capture none of it." And: "Computers needed to gather their own information by sensing the world for themselves" (Ashton).

The Internet of Things, then, is not merely an assemblage of smart devices but a drive to account for and connect all things, while reducing human intervention and oversight. It at once fosters a swelling technosensorium, where computers hear and smell "for themselves" and, at the same time, treats people with managerial indifference. Human users are understood to frustrate smartness through their errors and meaty slowness, even as they are imagined to be the beneficiaries or subjects of smart systems (e.g., as consumers, workers, citizens, criminals, etc.). People are at once central to the idea of the Internet of Things and, at the same time, their agency is peculiarly proscribed. Framed as user-agents or dependent variables, users are increasingly tracked, predicted, and reorganized like other objects. One is here reminded of ideas about capture or dataveillance—to be able to gather, store, and augment human actions, computers must institute habits and protocols (Agre 2003)—but also the need to track how ideas about digital surveillance are transformed by the platform economy. Digital-cognitive optimization both undergirds smartness initiatives and is largely elided by the universal claims of smartness discourse itself.

This is because the latter tends toward biopolitical scales—global, populations, and ubiquity—and erases actually existing people or communities in the name of idealized claims or calculations.

Debates about surveillance and capture inform much of the current thinking about how value and exploitation operate in the information economy—what scholars like Shoshana Zuboff have called *The Age of Surveillance Capitalism* (2019). Written for a broad audience and summarizing a number of recent transformations, Zuboff's analysis focuses on the ways that the tech economy turns human experience into raw materials and behavioral data. She notes that while a fraction of this data is used to improve products or services, "the rest are declared as a proprietary behavioral surplus, fed into advanced manufacturing processes known as 'machine intelligence,' and fabricated into prediction products that anticipate what you will do now, soon, and later." What's more, these predictive operations have generated a marketplace all their own—what Zuboff terms the "*behavioral futures markets*" (8).

Zuboff's formulation offers a useful summary of much popular and academic thinking about the data economy. But it also signals the limits of what we think we know about networked life. What's useful about such analyses is their understanding of how value is extracted from seemingly free platforms and labor. That is, we are now well beyond simple data mining and targeted advertising—or even the slogan "if you don't know what the product is, the product is you." Instead, such approaches theorize a speculative economy based on behavior modification that is profoundly unequal and deeply invested in using networked sensors to reorganize and financialize people and things. While this reorganization is often understood to be apolitical, offering technical solutions or efficiencies, surveillance capitalism, among similar critiques, distills the daily actions and platform monopolies driving contemporary forms of speculation and surplus.

One popular thread in this context links digital devices and networks to drug addiction, among similar habituations. From popular

anxieties about the internet's effects on our brains (Carr 2010)
to concerns about how Facebook's "dopamine-driven feedback
loops . . . are destroying how society works" (Palihapitiya 2017) to
the spread of neurobiological discourse lamenting "Dopamine,
Smartphones, and You" (Haynes 2018). The latter, a research blog
summarizing findings at Harvard Medical School, reports that
smartphone attachments result from the "hyper-social environments" they generate—a potential for connectivity many magni-
tudes greater than traditional social networks. "Although not as intense as hit of cocaine," the researcher Trevor Haynes summarizes,
"positive social stimuli will similarly result in a release of dopamine,
reinforcing whatever behavior preceded it," and rewiring our brains
in the process. Research in this vein frames human relationships to
smartphones as a battle over our time, habits, and the very routes
taken by neurotransmitters. The solution to these problems, the
works implies, is simply to put down our devices, turn off notifica-
tions, be mindful of time.

But beyond any neat computational interface or encounter, where
users are tracked, rewarded, or generate content lies another
diagram of networked life. If the tendency to focus on social media,
screens, and surveillance has emphasized certain human actions
or extensions, it has also overlooked other enmeshments between
humans and computers. In this way, technopharmacology can be
understood to reach beyond classical questions of consumption,
agency, sense making, or milieu. Instead it opens onto lesser
considered *intensities* or interiorizing trajectories—that is, processes of coming into the body that refuse familiar separations
between inside and outside or the boundedness of skin. Just as
networks consume human vitalities, so too do people *eat* or *ingest*
the network (Preciado 2013). Critical to this formulation is both
a commitment to human scales and politics *and* an investment
in nonhuman or planetary relations.[13] In this way humans are
active, not simply a ledger of actions; excitable, not merely raw
materials; infrastructures, not only user-participants. Building on
Susanna Paasonen's insistence on excitability and the "deeper

infrastructural dependencies" informing techno–human relations (see chapter 1), I argue that pharmacology animates our capacities to think, feel, and aspire in ways not accounted for by models of the data economy, logistical media, platform capitalism, and similar understandings of technoeconomic interpolation.

What I call the Internet of People and Things (IoPT) shores up a particular mode of human and nonhuman capture that is deeply invested in and extracted from performance enhancement and yet exceeds the isolated focus on the value of data. Instead we must continue to examine the shifting relations between "behavioral surplus" and data futures, on the one hand, and the forms of "surplus life" driving the bioeconomy, on the other (Cooper 2008; Vora 2015). These distinct surplus modalities pose tensions between *resilience* and *hyperbolic performance* at the center of smartness paradigms. If the former emphasizes crisis and adaptability—that is, the capacity to absorb shock and continue to function—the latter emphasizes not merely continued operability but the drive toward optimal effectiveness *beyond* existing constraints (including new forms of exhaustion, toxicity, and death on a human and planetary scale). This is not merely to describe a state of being *after equilibrium,* where the world is imagined as plastic and responsive to crisis, but rather to engage the manifold obligations shaping life *after optimization,* where so-called best practices and efficiencies amplify inequality and harm in the name of better futures (McKelvey and Neves 2021). In other words, crisis and optimization are mutually constitutive, just as they are unequally distributed.

I take my cue from what Melinda Cooper, in her discussion of biological speculation and accumulation, identifies as capital's "counterlogic"—that is, the simple fact that capital must always subtract from the surplus it creates. Of the transformations in *surplus life* brought about by the shift from industrial to postindustrial capitalism, Cooper writes:

> The difference [between the two] lies merely in their temporalities: while industrial production depletes the earth's

reserves of past organic life (carbon-based fossil fuels), postindustrial bioproduction needs to depotentialize the future possibilities of life, even while it puts them to work. This counterlogic is perhaps most visible in the use of patented sterilization technologies, where a plant's capacity to reproduce itself is both mobilized as a source of labor and deliberately curtailed, thus ensuring that it no longer reproduces "for free." But it is also endemic to the whole enterprise of capitalized bioproduction.

The friction between *depletion* and *depotentialization* is crucial to the work of resilience in our present conjuncture. No longer seeking equilibrium through medicine or risk mitigation—such as the economies of chronic health identified by Joseph Dumit (2012)—resilient bodies and technologies have reached a new impasse. They are now understood to be endlessly optimizable and, at the same time, to operate by proscribing future states. This normalizes a mode of vertical reproduction starting from the seeds a farmer must purchase and plant but not reuse, all the way to bioengineered foodstuffs or health supplements shipped to global markets. Owning, capturing, and modifying vital organisms now animates value extraction—including new and old forms of "biopiracy" (Shiva 2001)—where nothing produces "for free."

Cooper's surplus helps to demonstrate a basic claim of this chapter and our book: questioning the present requires a deeper engagement with data capitalism and pharmaceutical capitalism. This includes, as suggested above, the increasingly ordinary ways that stimulants like caffeine and nicotine, Ritalin and Adderall, Modafinil and nootropics, not to mention illegal narcotics, are enmeshed or *enfleshed* with smart technologies and computational networks. Understood to optimize and create new demands for focus, energy, productivity, and creativity, among other vitalities, these techno-pharmacologies are at once tied to a global rise in amphetamine-type stimulants (ATS) and technologized stimulations. Such concerns signal a continued de- and recomposing of the present and the planet that require new questions, methods, and focus areas.

**Intensions and the Political**

If *intensions*—material pathways into and through the body—are largely absent from contemporary media theory, they are also neglected by cultural understandings of medicine and other substances. As the anthropologist Asha Persson puts it: "It seems every aspect of the medical process has been critically analysed right up to the moment when drugs pass human lips and disappear down the oesophagus. After that, the story tends to become obscure, as if lost to the silent recesses of the body" (2004, 45). In her examination of HIV drugs and changing bodily appearance, Persson traces how drugs meet the "living flesh" and how bodies are "far from silent" (45–46). In this brief concluding section, I draw out a few implications of such insights for media theory, adding media technologies to the scene of biochemical ingestion.

In particular, I have been inspired by recent approaches to elemental media and their potential for engaging technology and pharmacology. To mention just two examples: John Durham Peter's *The Marvelous Clouds: Toward a Philosophy of Elemental Media* and Nicole Starosielski's "The Elements of Media Studies" exemplify an elemental turn that shifts and expands how we understand media's scale and scope. Peters describes this shift in focus as a move from figure to ground. He writes: "The elemental legacy of the media concept is fully relevant in a time when our most pervasive surrounding environment is technological and nature—from honeybees and dogs to corn and viruses, from the ocean floor to the atmosphere—is drenched with human manipulation" (2). In this way, he expands mediation to include the human-impacted natural world and those most basic of all elements: sea, earth, fire, and sky.

This historically rooted shift in our contemporary understanding of media brings atmospheric, environmental, and planetary dimensions and transformations to the center of current debates about technology. It is a line of thinking that is at once generative— including capturing the complex natural-artificiality of drugs, currents, and other optimizing supplements at issue here—and, as I have argued, is part of a larger set of assumptions that tends to understand media as outside, environmental, infrastructural, thingly. It is, to reiterate Peters's claim, a way of zooming out from figure to ground. While this orientation has invigorated media research, and no doubt remains fertile, it also drives a set of assumptions that may inhibit alternative trajectories and ways of knowing. What I have lightly termed the *intensions of (hu)man* is thus a call for a renewed focus on the body and bodily processes within and alongside elemental discourse, beginning with pharmaceutical practices. Probing technological and pharmacological pathways into and through the body helps us to thicken current elemental epistemologies in media studies and to chart alternative compositions of human and nonhuman worlds.

As Starosielski reminds us, attending the elements is quite useful for dissolving familiar boundaries between inner and outer, discrete and distributed, hard and molecular. Like drugs and other substances, "*elements* compose," and it matters which processes of composition we choose to emphasize in our searching and thinking. "Elements are not things." Instead, she continues, "Scholarship on media's elements has repeatedly shown that they are processual, dynamic, and intra-active" (2020, n.p.). It is this dynamism and intra-activity that matters here—both as a call for new directions for engaging media and animating the media imagination and as an approach attuned to the technopharmacological processes shaping contemporary economic, social, and political formations.

Consider what Margaret Morse, writing three decades ago, termed the "oral logic" of the information society in her essay "What Do Cyborg's Eat?" (1994, 88). Morse's essay draws on feminist cyborg interventions, including Donna Haraway's classic "Cyborg Manifesto," and avoids the later pitfalls identified by scholars like Katherine Hayles in her debunking of millennial understandings of information as the "code of the body," and thus entirely separable from it (1999, 1). Of this oral logic, Morse asks, "What do humans who want to become electronic eat?" She continues:

For we are no longer talking about metaphors or electronic prostheses that extend organic body functions (in the way Marshall McLuhan understands the media, for instance), or even about Frankensteinian reassemblage or Tin Man-like displacements of the organic body part by part. In this more *mechanical* sense, cyborgs with heart monitors, organ implants, and artificial limbs already walk the earth. The contemporary fantasy is rather how, if the organic body cannot be abandoned, it might be fused with electronic culture in what amounts to an *oral* logic of *incorporation.* (1994, 87)

No longer chiefly concerned with transcending the body, Morse, like Persson, draws our attention the material facts of human and nonhuman existence. Food and waste and muscle and skin jostle against heart monitors, implants, and more mundane electronic fusions. In this context, everyday practices of incorporation and absorption replace sci-fi fantasies, even as they must coexist with and integrate proliferating technical objects and processes.

Another prescient passage from Morse reflects on eating smart foods and drugs as a way to understand networked bodies in the 1990s. She writes:

Currently, when we want to introject cyborgs, "smart" drinks and drugs will have to do. Built along the analogy of smart appliances, houses, and bombs, the adjective *smart* attributes some degree of agency and, at times, of human subjectivity to the object world. "Smart" pill and powder cuisine consists of vitamins and/or drugs, laced at times with psychotropics and aimed directly for the brain. To the cyberpunk culinary imaginary, these chemicals are decidedly Utopian, a kind of lubricant or "tuneup" for wetware that breaks the blood-brain barrier, makes neurons fire faster, and encourages dendrite growth, not unlike the networks linking the electronic channels along which information flows. (89)

What's striking about Morse's meditation on smart bodies is how well it holds up in the present, despite its dated references. The description of smart foods, drinks, and drugs resonates strongly with the examples considered in this chapter. It underlines the importance of intensions, or incorporations as acts of mediation—the very processes through which bodies may emerge and merge, be truncated or thrive. My point in highlighting bodily and biological intersections is not to conflate intensions with processes of interiorization, nor to claim that metaphors of ingestion, inhalation and the like, offer a simple solution or remedy. Clearly there are other centripetal gestures—microbial, philosophical, ecological, and otherwise—that matter here. The simple suggestion is that the tendency to pursue outside forces, sites, and prostheses has overextended itself and now comes in the way of understanding important shifts in the technologized present. Attending pharmacological practices, like taking a pill or applying electrical current, is one modest way to reroute these affinities.

Finally, this is to return to Ruha Benjamin's speculative intervention, quoted in the epigraph. Drawing on her research into the social imagination of biotechnologies, Benjamin zeroes in on our contradictory and harmful commitments to individual transformation at the expense of wider social change. As she puts it, we must examine the peculiar faith currently invested in "biological regeneration" and ask why, if *our bodies can regenerate,* do we see *"our body politic as so utterly fixed?"* (2016, 3). This tension is central to the politics of smart technologies and cognitive enhancement, which supply endless applications for self-improvement while framing the social and planetary through the lens of crisis, apathy, and despair. In other words, frictions between resilience and optimization resonate far beyond specialized discourse. Benjamin's modest challenge is to generate new fictions and speculative methods that contest the larger fictions around us. If the tech and pharma industries spend billions to shape our sense of what is possible, then it is urgent both to understand these visions and to begin create our own. This is to ask: what forms of research and critique are needed to challenge the world picture articulated by smartness imperatives, technopharma platforms, and biotech imaginaries, especially to challenge the conceptual frameworks and political might that position their demands as norms? And how can we better attend the complex geopolitical intimacies and life-support systems that animate unequal optimization and extraction regimes across cities and continents? If a simple gesture of this book is to add pharmacology to existing understandings of networked technologies, it also suggests that our political critique and media theories must attend the larger networks of life and technics that constitute the present, including and beyond the human body.

## Notes

1    Elemental media is particularly interesting in this context. On the face of it, Peters's "sea, fire, sky, clouds, books, and God" (2015, 8) remain focused on the environment and are tied to understandings of nature, habitats, and atmospheres. But elemental media also focus meaning, infrastructure, and processes of composition. See also Starosielski (2019). I return to this line of thought in the conclusion.

2    Extension and externalization should not, of course, be seamlessly conflated. My interest is to underline both longstanding and contemporary ways of understanding media as external to, or extensions of, the body and to further signal how this tendency consolidates a certain common sense about what and where media *are*. These epistemological tendencies should not themselves be taken for hard categories (e.g. inside/outside). See also Lev Manovich's discussion of the "externalization of psyche" for a parallel analysis of the tendency to locate and understand mental states through their externalization in (historically available) media technologies and metaphors (Manovich 1995).

3    Here I both draw on an older usage of the term *intension* and coin a simple antonym for extension. The former draws on the definition of intension from logic, indicating "the internal quantity or content of a notion or concept, the sum of the attributes contained in it" (OED). Further, tracing intensions is not simply to call for a media "internalization" paradigm that parallels McLuhan's own commitment to prosthetics and external objects. Instead each are vectors in a web of life that must necessarily take human form and politics seriously without ceding its investments in nonhuman or planetary relations.

4    Stimulants and opiates should also be understood as part of the polypharmacy —the stacking of substances to achieve microstates, moods, and vitalities like focus, creativity, affability, confidence, rest, calm, and so on.

5    For a discussion of the complexity of opiate use in China's risky boom era, see Bartlett (2018). Further, the contemporary opium epidemic at once complicates

claims about the rise of stimulants and, at the same time, can be seen as a direct response to these cultures of speed, optimization, and risk.

6  Consider the history of cannabis use in India, for example (Chopra and Chopra 1957).

7  This mixture of new and old stimulants, everyday and experimental substances, cheap and expensive drugs/devices, and so on is crucial to my understanding of *smart drugs as a polypharmacy*. My point is not to call out nootropic supplements or costly devices as particularly new or impactful—though they certainly capture a certain ethos/ethics and often profit from traditional medicine or existing therapies—but to signal the continued growth and normalization of technological-pharmaceutical interventions in the everyday habits of living in much of the world.

8  Companies like JUUL, in the United States, and RELX, in the People's Republic of China, have thrived despite repeated setbacks regarding product safety, lack of regulations, and other issues related to public health, teen consumption, and deaths. See, for example, Yujie Xue, "China's Largest e-Cigarette Brand Relx to Study Health Effects of Vaping amid Regulatory Crackdowns," *South China Morning Post* (online), September 18, 2020, https://www.scmp.com/tech/science-research/article/3102028/chinas-largest-e-cigarette-brand-relx-study-health-effects. In contrast to the tentative success of e-cigarette companies in those markets, India banned the use of e-cigarettes in September 2019, citing concerns about safety and fear of a youth epidemic. See Sushmi Dey, "Fearing 'Epidemic among Kids, Young,' Govt Bans e-Cigarettes," *Times of India* (online), September 19, 2019, https://timesofindia.indiatimes.com/business/india-business/fearing-epidemic-among-kids-young-government-bans-e-cigarettes/articleshow/71192894.cms.

9  Formerly Nootrobox, HVMN has transformed its product line and rhetoric since I began to follow the company in 2017. Gone now is its sole focus on nootropic pills, including an entire section of the website focused on the science of nootropics for self-optimization. HVMN's current business model, while still selling supplements, focuses on keto nutrition, including food bars, collagen, and MCT powders, and the "Kickstarter keto kit." See https://hvmn.com/.

10  Since I began this research in 2017, Halo Sport has rebranded as Halo, and Halo Neuro, and expanded its product line to include sports drinks, among other things. For an overview of the "science," see https://www.haloneuro.com/pages/science. As of the summer of 2021, the product has been discontinued. Among the reasons for this are the proliferation of similar devices and a crowded marketplace. See Neves and Chia's future work on wearable devices like Apollo, NeoRhythm, and BrainTap (an essay in progress for a special issue of the *Media Theory* journal on "pharmacologies of media").

11  There are thousands of such sites, ranging from individual users to community and corporate threads. See, for example, Quantified Self (https://quantifiedself.com/), subreddits dedicated to Transcranial Direct Current Stimulation (https://www.reddit.com/r/tDCS/) or nootropics (https://www.reddit.com/r/Nootropics/)

or the Facebook group for NeoRythm (https://www.facebook.com/omnipemf/), a popular neurotech wearable.

12    "Still Zapping My Brain. DIY tDCS Volume Two," YouTube (2012), https://www.youtube.com/watch?v=ORvXUQuRs8c.

13    I have been asked whether my commitment to the human in this chapter relies on a set of assumptions about a unified subject that can be breached or rearranged by drugs or technology. In other words, have I merely upheld McLuhan's extensions from a different perspective? My answer to this question is yes and no. In my view, human politics remain central but insufficient to address the technopharmacological challenges posed by the present. Among similar interventions, I here follow Dipesh Chakrabarty's recent work on climate change, the planetary, and the category of the human. He writes: "Posthumanism by itself cannot address the political. Any theory of politics adequate to the planetary crisis humans face today would have to begin from the same old premise of securing human life but now ground itself in a new philosophical anthropology, that is in a new understanding of the changing place of humans in the web of life and in the connected but different histories of the globe and the planet" (2019, 30).

## References

Agre, Philip. 2003. "Surveillance and Capture: Two Models of Privacy." In *The New Media Reader*. Ed. Noah Wardrip-Fruin and Nick Monfort, 737–59. Cambridge, Mass.: MIT Press.

Ashton, Kevin. 2015. "Beginning the Internet of Things." Blog: https://www.howtofly ahorse.com/beginning-the-internet-of-things/.

Andreas, Peter. 2020. "The World War II 'Wonder Drug' That Never Left Japan." *Zocalo,* January 8. https://www.zocalopublicsquare.org/2020/01/08/the-world-war-ii -wonder-drug-that-never-left-japan/ideas/essay/.

Bartlett, Nicholas. 2018. "The Ones Who Struck Out: Entrepreneurialism, Heroin Addiction, and Historical Obsolescence in Reform Era China." *positions: east asia critique* 26, no. 3: 423-449.

Battleday, R. M. and A.-K. Brem. 2015. "Modafinil for Cognitive Neuroenhancement in Healthy Non-Sleep-Deprived Subjects: A Systematic Review." *European Neuropsychopharmacology* 25:1865–81.

Benjamin, Ruha. 2016. "Racial Fictions, Biological Facts: Expanding the Sociological Imagination through Speculative Methods." *Catalyst: Feminism, Theory, Technoscience* 2, no. 2: 1–28.

Beyes, Timon, Lisa Conrad, and Reinhold Martin. 2019. *Organize.* Lüneburg and Minneapolis: meson press and University of Minnesota Press.

Brown, Wendy. 2016. "Selling Democracy: Part One of the Way of Neoliberalism" Interview with Doug Storm. *Interchange.* October 18. https://wfhb.org/news/ interchange-selling-democracy-part-one-of-the-way-of-neoliberalism/.

Carr, Nicholas. 2010. *The Shallows: What the Internet Is Doing to Your Brain.* New York: W.W. Norton.

Chakrabarty, Dipesh. 2019. "The Planet: An Emergent Humanist Category." *Critical*
    *Inquiry* 46: 1–31.

Chatterjee, Anjan. 2004. "Cosmetic Neurology: The Controversy over Enhancing
    Movement, Mentation, and Mood," *Neurology* 63, no. 6: 968–74.

Chopra, I.C. and R.N. Chopra. 1957. "The Use of Cannabis Drugs in India." United
    Nations Office on Drugs and Crime Bulletin: 4–29. https://www.unodc.org/unodc/
    en/data-and-analysis/bulletin/bulletin_1957-01-01_1_page003.html.

Chun, Wendy Hui Kyong. 2016. *Updating to Remain the Same: Habitual New Media.*
    Cambridge, Mass.: MIT Press.

Cooper, Melinda. 2008. *Life as Surplus: Biotechnology and Capitalism in the Neoliberal
    Era.* Seattle: University of Washington Press.

Crary, Jonathan. 2014. *24/7.* New York: Verso.

Dance, Amber. 2016. "A Dose of Intelligence." *Nature* 531 (March 3): S2–S3.

Derrida, Jacques. 1981. *Dissemination.* Trans. Barbara Johnson. London: The Athlone
    Press.

Dikötter, Frank, Lars Laamann, and Zhou Xun. 2004. *Narcotic Culture: A History of
    Drugs in China.* Chicago: University of Chicago Press.

Dumit, Joseph. 2012. *Drugs for Life: How Pharmaceutical Companies Define Our Health.*
    Durham, N.C.: Duke University Press, 2012.

Ehrenreich, Barbara, and John Ehrenreich. 2013. "Death of a Yuppie Dream: The
    Rise and Fall of the Professional Managerial Class." New York: Rosa Luxemburg
    Siftung.

Halpern, Orit, Robert Mitchell, and Bernard Dionysius Geoghegan. 2017. "The Smart-
    ness Mandate: Notes toward a Critique," *Grey Room* 68 (Summer): 106–29.

Han Minglian. 2011. "The Appeal of Marshall McLuhan in Contemporary China."
    *Canadian Social Science* 7, no. 3: 1–6.

Harbeck, Rebecca. 2019. "The Evolution of China's Coffee Industry." *US-China Today,*
    June 28. https://uschinatoday.org/features/2019/06/28/the-evolution-of-chinas
    -coffee-industry/.

Hayles, N. Katherine. 2001. *How We Became Posthuman: Virtual Bodies in Cybernetics,
    Literature, and Informatics.* Chicago: University of Chicago Press.

Haynes, Trevor. 2018. "Dopamine, Smartphones & You: The Battle for Your Time."
    *Science in the News* blog. https://sitn.hms.harvard.edu/flash/2018/dopamine-smart
    phones-battle-time/.

Kember, Sarah, and Joanna Zylinska. 2014. *Life after New Media: Mediation as Vital
    Process.* Cambridge, Mass.: MIT Press.

Kittler, Friedrich A. 1999. *Gramophone, Film, Typewriter.* Trans. Geoffrey Winthrop-
    Young and Michael Wutz. Palo Alto, Calif.: Stanford University Press.

Leroi-Gourhan, André. 1993 [1964]. *Gesture and Speech.* Trans. Anna Bostock Berger.
    Cambridge, Mass.: MIT Press.

Manovich, Lev. 1995. "From the Externalization of the Psyche to the Implantation of
    Technology." http://manovich.net/index.php/projects/from-the-externalization
    -of-the-psyche-to-the-implantation-of-technology.

McKelvey, Fenwick and Joshua Neves. 2021. "Introduction: Optimization and its
    Discontents." *Review of Communication* 21, no. 2: 95–112.

McLuhan, Marshall. 1994 [1964]. *Understanding Media: The Extensions of Man.* Cambridge, Mass.: MIT Press.

Mitchell, W. J. T. and Mark B. N. Hansen, Eds. 2010. *Critical Terms for Media Studies.* Chicago: University of Chicago Press.

Morris, Alex. 2016. "The Pill Freaks of Silicon Valley." *New York Magazine.* https://nymag.com/intelligencer/2016/10/nootrobox-wants-to-hack-your-brain.html.

Morse, Margaret. 1994. "What Do Cyborgs Eat? Oral Logic in an Information Society." *Discourse* 16, no. 3: 86–123.

Mukherjee, Rahul. 2020. *Radiant Infrastructures: Media, Environment, and Cultures of Uncertainty.* Durham, N.C.: Duke University Press.

Neves, Joshua. 2020. "Social Media and the Social Question: Speculations on Risk Media Society." In *The Routledge Companion to Media and Risk,* Ed. Bhaskar Sarkar and Bishnupriya Ghosh, 347–61. New York: Routledge.

Palihapitiya, Chamath. 2017. "Founder and CEO Social Capital, on Money as an Instrument of Change." Stanford Graduate School of Business YouTube channel. https://www.youtube.com/watch?v=PMotykw0Sik.

Partridge, Bradley. 2012. "Students and 'Smart Drugs': Empirical Research Can Shed Light on Enhancement Enthusiasm." *Asian Bioethics Review* 4, no. 2: 310–19.

Persson, Asha. 2004. "Incorporating *Pharmakon:* HIV, Medicine, and Body Shape Change." *Body & Society* 10, no. 4: 45–67.

Peters, John Durham. 2015. *The Marvelous Clouds: Toward a Philosophy of Elemental Media.* Chicago: University of Chicago Press.

Pine, Jason. 2007. "Economy of Speed: The New Narco-Capitalism." *Public Culture* 19, no. 2: 357–66.

Pine, Jason. 2019. *The Alchemy of Meth: A Decomposition.* Minneapolis: University of Minnesota Press.

Preciado, Paul B. 2013. *Testo Junkie: Sex, Drugs, and Biopolitics in the Pharmapornographic Era.* New York: The Feminist Press.

Race, Kane. 2015. "'Party and Play': Online Hook-Up Devices and the Emergence of PNP Practices among Gay Men." *Sexualities* 18, no. 3: 253–75.

Rinella, Michael A. 2010. *Pharmakon: Plato, Drug Culture, and Identity in Ancient Athens.* New York: Lexington Books.

Sato, Akihiko. 2008. "Methamphetamine Use in Japan after the Second World War: Transformation of Narratives." *Contemporary Drug Problems* 35:717–43.

Schivelbush, Wolfgang. 1992. *Tastes of Paradise: A Social History of Spices, Stimulants, and Intoxicants.* Trans. David Jacobson. New York: Vintage Books.

Shiva, Vandana. 2001. *Protect or Plunder?: Understanding Intellectual Property Rights.* London: ZED Books.

Smith, Matthew. 2017. "Hyperactive around the World? The History of ADHD in Global Perspective." *Social History of Medicine* 30, no. 4: 767–87.

Starosielski, Nicole. 2019. "The Elements of Media Studies." *Media+Environment* 1, no. 1: https://mediaenviron.org/article/10780-the-elements-of-media-studies.

Steinberg, Marc. 2017. "McLuhan a Prescription Drug: Actionable Theory and Advertising Industries." In *Media Theory in Japan,* Ed. Marc Steinberg and Alex Zahlten, 131–50. Durham, N.C.: Duke University Press.

Stiegler, Bernard. 1998. *Technics and Time, 1: The Fault of Epimetheus.* Trans. Richard Beardsworth and George Collins. Stanford, Calif.: Stanford University Press.

Vora, Kalindi. 2015. *Life Support: Biocapital and the New History of Outsourced Labor.* Durham, N.C.: Duke University Press.

Wolkoff, David A.1997. "Methamphetamine Abuse: An Overview for Health Care Professionals." *Hawaii Medical Journal* 56: 34–36.

Wurzman, Rachel, Roy H. Hamilton, Alvaro Pascual-Leone, and Michael D. Fox. 2016. "An Open Letter Concerning Do-It-Yourself Users of Transcranial Direct Current Stimulation." *Annals of Neurology* 80, no. 1: 1–4.

Zhang Shaoxiang. 2015. "Digital Medicine: An Exciting Field of Medical Sciences." *Digital Medicine* 1, no. 1: 1–2.

Zuboff, Shoshana. 2019. *The Age of Surveillance Capitalism: The Fight for a Human Future at the New Frontier of Power.* New York: Public Affairs.

## Authors

**Aleena Chia** is lecturer in media, communications, and cultural studies at Goldsmiths, University of London, where she researches creative cultures in game development and computational wellness.

**Joshua Neves** is associate professor of film studies at Concordia University, and author of *Underglobalization: Beijing's Media Urbanism and the Chimera of Legitimacy.*

**Susanna Paasonen** is professor of media studies at the University of Turku, Finland, and author of *Dependent, Distracted, Bored: Affective Formations in Networked Media.*

**Ravi Sundaram** is professor at the Centre for the Study of Developing Societies (CSDS), Delhi. He is author of *Pirate Modernity: Delhi's Media Urbanism* and editor of *No Limits: Media Studies from India.*